Environmental Health Criteria 115

2-METHOXYETHANOL, 2-ETHOXYETHANOL, AND THEIR ACETATES

Published under the joint sponsorship of the United Nations Environment Programme, the International Labour Organisation, and the World Health Organization

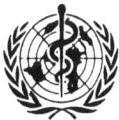

World Health Organization
Geneva, 1990

The **International Programme on Chemical Safety (IPCS)** is a joint venture of the United Nations Environment Programme, the International Labour Organisation, and the World Health Organization. The main objective of the IPCS is to carry out and disseminate evaluations of the effects of chemicals on human health and the quality of the environment. Supporting activities include the development of epidemiological, experimental laboratory, and risk-assessment methods that could produce internationally comparable results, and the development of manpower in the field of toxicology. Other activities carried out by the IPCS include the development of know-how for coping with chemical accidents, coordination of laboratory testing and epidemiological studies, and promotion of research on the mechanisms of the biological action of chemicals.

WHO Library Cataloguing in Publication Data

2-Methoxyethanol, 2-ethoxyethanol, and their acetates.

(Environmental health criteria ; 115)

1. Ethylene glycols - adverse effects   2. Ethylene glycols - toxicity
I. Series

ISBN 92 4 157115 2   (NLM Classification: QV 633)
ISSN 0250-863X

Printed in Finland
90/8558 — Vammala — 5000

CONTENTS

ENVIRONMENTAL HEALTH CRITERIA FOR
2-METHOXYETHANOL, 2-ETHOXYETHANOL,
AND THEIR ACETATES

4

WHO TASK GROUP ON ENVIRONMENTAL HEALTH CRITERIA FOR 2-METHOXYETHANOL, 2-ETHOXYETHANOL, AND THEIR ACETATES

Members

Dr W. Denkhaus, Institute for Occupational and Social Medicine, University of Mainz, Mainz, Federal Republic of Germany

Dr R.J. Fielder, Medical TEH Division, Department of Health, Hannibal House, Elephant and Castle, London, United Kingdom

Dr B. Gilbert, Company for the Development of Technology Transfer (CODETEC), Cidade Universitaria, Campinas, Brazil *(Vice-Chairman)*

Dr B. Hardin, Division of Standards Development and Technology Transfer, National Institute for Occupational Safety and Health, Cincinnati, Ohio, USA

Dr M. Ikeda, Department of Public Health, Kyoto University Faculty of Medicine, Kyoto, Japan *(Chairman)*

Dr S.K. Kashyap, National Institute of Occupational Health, Ahmedabad, India

Dr L. Rosenstein, Office of Toxic Substances, US Environmental Protection Agency, Washington DC, USA

Dr J. Sokal, Institute of Occupational Medicine, Division of Industrial Toxicology, Lodz, Poland

Dr H. Veulemans, Laboratory for Occupational Hygiene, Department of Occupational Medicine, University of Leuven, Leuven, Belgium

Representatives of other Organizations

Dr K. Miller, International Commission on Occupational Health, British Industrial Biological Research Association, Carshalton, Surrey, United Kingdom

Observers

Dr A. Cicolella, Institut National de Recherche et de Sécurité, Vandoeuvre, France

Secretariat

Dr G. Becking, International Programme on Chemical Safety, Interregional Research Unit, World Health Organization, Research Triangle Park, North Carolina, USA *(Secretary)*

Dr H. Teitelbaum, US Environmental Protection Agency, Office of Toxic Substances, Washington DC, USA *(Rapporteur)*

NOTE TO READERS OF THE CRITERIA DOCUMENTS

Every effort has been made to present information in the criteria documents as accurately as possible without unduly delaying their publication. In the interest of all users of the environmental health criteria documents, readers are kindly requested to communicate any errors that may have occurred to the Manager of the International Programme on Chemical Safety, World Health Organization, Geneva, Switzerland, in order that they may be included in corrigenda, which will appear in subsequent volumes.

* * *

A detailed data profile and a legal file can be obtained from the International Register of Potentially Toxic Chemicals, Palais des Nations, 1211 Geneva 10, Switzerland (Telephone No. 7988400 or 7985850).

ENVIRONMENTAL HEALTH CRITERIA FOR
2-METHOXYETHANOL, 2-ETHOXYETHANOL, AND
THEIR ACETATES

A WHO Task Group on Environmental Health Criteria for 2-Methoxyethanol, 2-Ethoxyethanol, and their Acetates met at the British Industrial Biological Research Association (BIBRA), Surrey, United Kingdom, from 4 to 7 April 1989. The meeting was sponsored by the United Kingdom Department of Health and Social Services. Dr S.D. Gangoli, Director, BIBRA, welcomed the participants on behalf of the host institution, and Dr G.C. Becking opened the meeting on behalf of the three co-operating organizations of the IPCS (ILO/UNEP/WHO). The Task Group reviewed and revised the draft document and made an evaluation of the risks for humans and the environment from exposure to these four glycol ethers.

The first and second drafts of this document were prepared by Dr H. TEITELBAUM, US Environmental Protection Agency, Washington DC, USA.

The efforts of all who helped in the preparation and finalization of the document are gratefully acknowledged. Dr G. Becking and Dr P.G. Jenkins, both members of the IPCS Central Unit, were responsible for the overall scientific content and technical editing, respectively.

ABBREVIATIONS

ADH	alcohol dehydrogenase
EAA	ethoxyacetic acid
ECG	electrocardiogram
2-EE	2-ethoxyethanol
2-EEA	2-ethoxyethyl acetate
GC-FID	gas chromatography with flame ionization detector
HPLC	high performance liquid chromatography
LOEL	lowest-observed-effect level
MAA	methoxyacetic acid
2-ME	2-methoxyethanol
2-MEA	2-methoxyethyl acetate
NIOSH	National Institute for Occupational Safety and Health (USA)
NOEL	no-observed-effect level
ODC	ornithine decarboxylase
OSHA	Occupational Safety and Health Administration (USA)
PCB	polychlorinated biphenyl
SCE	sister chromatid exchange
TWA	time-weighted average
UDS	unscheduled DNA synthesis

1. SUMMARY AND CONCLUSIONS

1.1   Identity, Physical and Chemical Properties, Analytical Methods

This monograph considers only the methyl and ethyl ethers of ethylene glycol, i.e. 2-methoxyethanol (2-ME) and 2-ethoxyethanol (2-EE), and their respective acetate esters, 2-methoxyethyl acetate (2-MEA) and 2-ethoxyethyl acetate (2-EEA). These four compounds are all stable, colourless, flammable liquids with a mild ethereal odour and are all miscible with (or in the case of 2-EEA very soluble in) water and miscible with a large number of organic solvents.

Analytical methods are available for the detection of these glycol ethers or their metabolites in various media (air, water, blood, and urine). They often employ adsorption or extraction procedures to concentrate the sample, followed by gas chromatographic analysis. Using gas or high performance liquid chromatography, 2-methoxyacetic acid (MAA) and 2-ethoxyacetic acid (EAA), (metabolites of 2-ME and 2-EE) can be measured in urine, usually after derivatization, at concentrations between 5 and 100 μg/ml.

1.2   Sources of Human and Environmental Exposure

The four glycol ethers reviewed are all produced by the reaction of ethylene oxide with the appropriate alcohol, followed, when required, by esterification with ethanoic acid.

Data for world production of these glycol ethers are not available. However, the combined annual production in Western Europe, USA, and Japan is approximately 79 x 10^3 tonnes of 2-ME and 205 x 10^3 tonnes of 2-EE. A large proportion is used in the coatings industry (paints, stains, and lacquers) and as solvents for printing inks, resins and dyes, and home and industrial cleaners. They are also used as anti-icing additives in hydraulic fluids and jet fuel.

1.3 Environmental Transport, Distribution, and Transformation

The solubility of these glycol ethers in water and their relatively low vapour pressure could result in their build-up in water in the absence of degradation. However, degradation by microorganisms in soil, sewage sludge, and water appears to prevent this possibility.

Atmospheric emissions resulting from the use of glycol ethers as evaporative solvents result in the greatest environmental exposure. In the general environment, photolytic degradation appears to be rapid, and levels below 0.0007 mg/m^3 (2 x 10^{-4} ppm) would be expected.

Under aerobic conditions glycol ethers are degraded rapidly by microorganisms to carbon dioxide and water, whereas under anaerobic conditions methane and carbon dioxide are the major end-products.

1.4 Environmental Levels and Human Exposures

The use of glycol ethers can result in significant widespread emissions to the environment. There is particular concern for direct human exposure in industry, in small work-shops, and during home use of products containing glycol ethers. Occupational exposure values of < 0.1 mg/m^3 to > 150 mg/m^3 have been reported. Significant exposure could occur to users of consumer products but no data are available.

In addition to exposure from airborne glycol ethers, humans may be exposed dermally. Blood analyses confirm rapid absorption by this route, which may contribute more than airborne exposure to the total body burden.

1.5 Kinetics and Metabolism

All four glycol ethers have been shown to be readily absorbed through the skin, lungs, and gastrointestinal tract. The highest levels detected in distribution studies on 2-ME in pregnant mice were in the maternal liver, blood, and gastrointestinal tract, and in the placenta, yolk sac, and numerous embryonic structures.

The metabolic transformation of 2-ME gives two primary metabolites: MAA and 2-methoxyacetyl glycine. Metabolism to carbon dioxide represents a secondary, minor route. The conversion in plasma of 2-ME to MAA is rapid, with a half-life of 0.6 h in rats, but the excretion of MAA is slow, with a half-life of about 20 h in the rat and 77 h in man.

In laboratory animals, administration of 2-EE led to the production of EAA and 2-ethoxyacetyl glycine, EAA being the major metabolite appearing in the presumptive target organ, the testes. In a human study using 2-EEA, a similar metabolic pathway was seen, the acetate being hydrolyzed first to 2-EE and subsequently oxidized to EAA. The resultant EAA was excreted with an estimated half-life of 21-42 h. Experimental work suggests that the retention or *accumulation* of metabolites could be toxicologically significant assuming that these metabolites are responsible for the observed target-organ toxicity.

1.6 Effects on Organisms in the Environment

The toxicity of 2-ME and 2-EE to microorganisms and aquatic animals appears to be low. For microorganisms, the lethal concentration in the medium is greater than 2%. Growth inhibition of green algae by 2-ME was noted at 10^4 mg/litre and of cyanobacteria (blue-green algae) at 100 mg per litre. The acute toxicity of 2-EE is very low for arthropods (LC_{50} > 4 g/litre) and freshwater fish (LC_{50} > 10 g per litre). The glycol ether acetates (2-MEA and 2-EEA) are far more toxic to fish. The LC_{50} of 2-EEA for fathead minnows is 46 mg/litre and that of 2-MEA for tidewater silverfish and bluegills is 45 mg/litre. There have been no long-term studies.

1.7 Effects on Experimental Animals and *In Vitro* Test Systems

1.7.1 Systemic toxicity

The toxicity of 2-ME and 2-EE to experimental animals has been much more widely studied than that of 2-MEA and 2-EEA.

2-ME and 2-EE and their acetates have similar lethalities after single exposures and they show low acute lethality whether exposure is via the dermal, oral, or inhalation route. Oral LD_{50} values for a variety of species range between 900 and 3400 mg/kg body weight for 2-ME, 1400 and 5500 mg/kg for 2-EE, 1250 and 3930 mg/kg for 2-MEA, and 1300 and 5100 mg/kg for 2-EEA. Inhalation LC_{50} values of 4603 mg/m^3 (2-ME) and 6698 mg/m^3 (2-EE) have been reported in mice.

Only limited data on skin and eye irritation or on the sensitization potential of these glycol ethers in animals is available. It would appear that they are not irritating to the skin, but that they can cause eye irritation. No skin irritation or skin sensitization has been reported in humans in spite of extensive exposures.

Short-term inhalation exposure (up to 90 days) of experimental animals to high concentrations (> 9313 mg 2-ME/m^3 and > 1450 mg 2-EE/m^3) has been shown to lead to adverse effects on blood parameters, the nervous system, and testes, thymus, kidney, liver, and lung. At lower exposure levels, effects are observed on the haemopoietic system and testes. For example, rats exposed by inhalation to 2-ME for 13 weeks at levels between 93 and 930 mg/m^3 exhibited reduced packed cell volume and white blood cell, haemoglobin, platelet, and serum protein concen-trations at the highest dose only, while similarly exposed rabbits had decreased thymus size, in addition to the decreased blood parameters, at 930 mg/m^3. 2-EE exhibited similar but less severe effects in rats and rabbits when animals were exposed for 13 weeks at a level of 1450 mg/m^3. No data are available from long-term studies.

1.7.2   Carcinogenicity and mutagenicity

The mutagenicity of 2-ME has been investigated in a range of *in vitro* systems using bacteria and mammalian cells. Although most studies yielded negative results, there were reports of positive mutagenicity results at very high 2-ME concentrations in CHO cells when investi-gated for chromosome aberration (at 6830 µg/ml or more) and sister chromatid exchange (3170 µg/ml or more). However, *in vivo* studies for chromosome aberrations and micronuclei were negative. Only very limited information on the mutagenic potential of 2-EE is available, and there are no carcinogenicity data for these glycol ethers.

1.7.3 Male reproductive system

The effect of 2-ME on the male reproductive system has been intensively investigated following both oral and inhalation exposure in rodents. Degenerative changes in the germinal epithelium of the seminiferous tubules were consistently noted. Similar effects were seen with 2-EE but at somewhat higher dose levels.

Oral dosing of rats with 2-ME for 1-11 days resulted in a dose-related decrease in sperm count and changes in sperm motility and morphology at dose levels of 100 mg/kg body weight or more. Marked histological damage was seen in the testes at autopsy. The no-observed-effect level (NOEL) was 50 mg/kg. Reduced fertility was still evident 8 weeks after exposure to 200 mg/kg. Similar effects were seen at dose levels of 500 mg 2-EE/kg or more, given for up to 11 days, the NOEL for 11-day treatment being 250 mg/kg. However, when sperm reserves were depleted by repeated mating, some reduction in sperm counts was seen at the lowest dose investigated (150 mg/kg). Fertility studies following a single oral dose of 250 mg 2-ME/kg or more revealed complete sterility in both rats and mice at 5 weeks post dosing, some decrease in fertility being seen at 125 mg/kg.

When the inhalation route was investigated, similar degenerative changes in the testes were seen with 2-ME. Effects were observed following a single exposure (4 h) to 1944 mg/m^3 or more but not to 933 mg/m^3. NOEL values were 311 mg/m^3 in rats following exposure for 13 weeks (6 h/day, 5 day/week) and 933 mg/m^3 (6 h/day) in mice following exposure on 9 occasions over 11 days. Exposure of rabbits to 2-ME for 13 weeks (6 h/day, 5 days/week) resulted in marked effects on the testes at 311 mg/m^3 or more; marginal effects were seen at 93 mg/m^3, and a NOEL was not identified.

1.7.4 Developmental toxicity

Developmental toxicity has been observed in several species of laboratory animals following exposure by all routes of administration, i.e. oral, inhalation, and dermal. 2-ME produced teratogenic effects in mice, rats, rabbits, and monkeys. 2-EE and 2-EEA were teratogenic in rats and rabbits. Although 2-MEA has not been tested for developmental toxicity, metabolic profiles (see section 6) suggest that it is reasonable to expect that 2-MEA would have a toxicity similar to that of 2-ME.

The widest range of dose/response data (doses of 31.25 to 1000 mg/kg per day) is available for 2-ME. In this gavage study using mice, (2-ME was administered on days 7 to 14 of gestation), the NOEL for maternal toxicity was 125 mg/kg per day. However, malformations were observed at 62.5 mg/kg per day and skeletal variations at 31.25 mg/kg per day. A NOEL for developmental toxicity was not reported. In single-dose studies, mice were treated with 2-ME by gavage on gestation day 11; 100 mg/kg was not fetotoxic, while 175 mg/kg produced digit defects without other signs of maternal or fetal toxicity. Cardiovascular defects and ECG abnormalities were observed in neonatal rats following treatment on days 7 to 13 of gestation with 25 mg/kg per day. Since that was the lowest dose tested, this study yielded no developmental NOEL (maternal toxicity was not observed at that dose). Similarly, no NOEL for developmental toxicity could be determined when monkeys were treated by gavage with 2-ME at 0.16, 0.32, or 0.47 mmol/kg per day on days 20 to 45 of gestation.

Fetotoxicity in mice and rats and malformations in rabbits were observed following exposure by inhalation to 2-ME at 156 mg/m^3. For all three species, the NOEL for developmental effects was 31 mg/m^3. However, behavioural and neurochemical alterations were seen in the offspring of rats exposed to 78 mg 2-ME/m^3 on days 7-13 or 14-20 of gestation.

Following inhalation exposure of rats (743 mg/m^3) and rabbits (589 mg/m^3), 2-EE was found to be teratogenic (in the presence of slight maternal toxicity). Another study reported fetotoxicity but no malformations in rats exposed to 184 or 920 mg 2-EE/m^3, and in rabbits exposed to 644 mg 2-EE/m^3. NOEL values for developmental effects were 37 mg/m^3 for rats and 184 mg/m^3 for rabbits. Behavioural and neurochemical alterations were seen in the offspring of rats exposed to 368 mg 2-EE/m^3 on days 7-13 or 14-20 of gestation.

Rats treated by dermal application of 0.25 ml undiluted 2-EE (four times daily on gestation days 7-16) exhibited marked fetotoxicity and a high incidence of malformation in the absence of maternal toxicity. Similar effects were noted following 2-EEA treatment of rats, using the same protocol, at an equimolar dose (0.35 ml, four times daily).

Inhalation exposure of rabbits to 2-EEA on gestation days 6-18 produced teratogenic responses at 2176 mg/m^3 and 544 mg/m^3 in two different studies, the developmental NOEL values in these two studies being 135 mg/m^3 and 270 mg/m^3. Exposure of rats to 2-EEA on days 6-15 of gestation produced fetotoxicity at 540 mg/m^3 and malformation at 1080 mg/m^3. The developmental NOEL was 170 mg/m^3.

1.8 Effects on man

Information on the toxic effects of these four glycol ethers on humans is limited. The results from the few case reports and workplace epidemiological studies are consistent with the adverse effects seen in experimental animals. No reports quantifying general population exposure and health effects have been found.

In two non-fatal cases of poisoning by ingestion of 100 ml 2-ME, the predominant signs and symptoms were nausea, vertigo, cyanosis, tachycardia, hyperventilation, and metabolic acidosis, with some evidence of renal failure. Similar but less severe symptoms were found in a person ingesting 40 ml 2-EE. In a fatal poisoning resulting from the ingestion of 400 ml 2-ME, postmortem findings showed acute haemorrhagic gastritis, fatty degeneration of the liver, and degenerative changes in renal tubules.

Repeated exposure of workers to 2-ME and 2-EE, in addition to other solvents, resulted in anaemia, leucopenia, general weakness, and ataxia. No reliable estimation of exposure was made in many of these reported studies. Haematological effects of glycol ethers on humans have been documented and the development of macrocytic anaemia in a worker exposed to 2-ME (average 105 mg/m^3), along with other solvents, has been described.

Bone marrow toxicity has been reported in workers exposed dermally to 2-ME, and immunological effects have been noted in workers following prolonged exposure (8-35 years) to 2-ME and 2-EE (mean exposures being 6.1 mg/m^3 and 4.8 mg/m^3, respectively).

Epidemiological studies of workers exposed to 2-ME and 2-EE have shown some evidence of adverse effect on the male reproductive system, with an increased frequency of reduced sperm counts. Exposure to 2-EE (37 workers) at levels up to 88.5 mg/m^3 led to change in semen indices. Among 73 workers exposed to 2-ME (up to 17.7 mg/m^3) and 2-EE (up to 80.5 mg/m^3), there was an increased frequency of reduced sperm counts and also evidence of haematological effects when exposures (TWA) were 2.6 mg/m^3 for 2-ME and 9.9 mg/m^3 for 2-EE.

The adverse effects noted in humans exposed occupationally are consistent with those noted in experimental animals. However, due to deficiencies in exposure assessments and to mixed exposures, no dose-response relationships can be determined.

1.9 Conclusions

Many people may be exposed to these four glycol ethers at levels comparable to industrial levels through the use of consumer and trade products. Significant occupational exposure may occur both through inhalation and skin absorption. Limited measurements of air levels in the workplace range from < 0.1 mg/m^3 to > 150 mg/m^3.

Both 2-ME and 2-EE demonstrate low toxicity to micro-organisms and aquatic species. No data exist to ascertain the potential for adverse effects on environmental species from long-term exposure.

In rats, the NOEL in acute studies for testicular effects was 933 mg 2-ME/m^3, and the NOEL for repeated exposure was 311 mg/m^3. In repeated exposure studies using the most sensitive species, the rabbit, a clear effect was detected at 311 mg/m^3, whereas at 93 mg/m^3 there was a marginal effect (1 in 5 animals). Evidence from studies on men exposed occupationally to 2-ME and 2-EE indicates that these glycol ethers can produce testicular toxicity in humans.

Developmental toxicity has been observed in all species (mice, rats, and rabbits exposed to 2-ME at 156 mg/m^3 or more. The NOEL for all three species was 31 mg/m^3. Behavioural and neurochemical alterations in rats followed *in utero* exposure to 78 mg/m^3, no NOEL being identified. 2-EE and 2-EEA were slightly less potent. Developmental effects were observed in rats and rabbits following exposure to 2-EE at 368 mg/m^3 or more. These effects were slight in rats exposed to 184 mg 2-EE/m^3, but 37 mg/m^3 was a clear NOEL for both rats and rabbits.

Haematological effects are produced by these glycol ethers in mice, rat, rabbits, dogs, hamsters, and guinea-pigs. This agrees with haematological effects reported in some of the limited number of studies of industrial workers exposed repeatedly to 2-EE and/or 2-ME. In repeated-exposure animal studies, the NOEL was 93 mg 2-ME/m^3 in rabbits and 368 mg 2-EE/m^3 in rats and rabbits. No data have been found to evaluate quantitatively the haematological effects that follow acute exposure.

2. IDENTITY, PHYSICAL AND CHEMICAL PROPERTIES, ANALYTICAL METHODS

2.1   Identity

The four glycol ethers discussed in this monograph, i.e. 2-methoxyethanol (2-ME), 2-methoxyethyl acetate (2-MEA), 2-ethoxyethanol (2-EE), and 2-ethoxyethyl acetate (2-EEA), are stable flammable liquids with a slight odour at normal room temperature and pressure. Their structural formulae are:

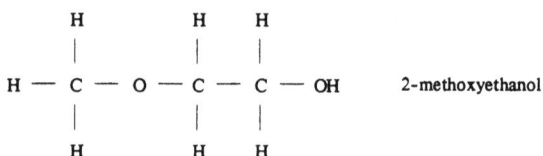

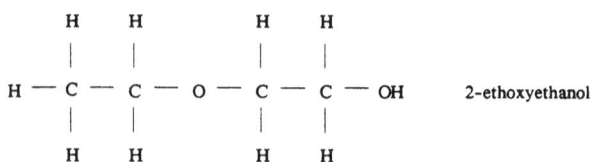

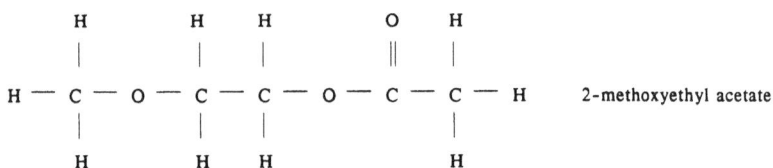

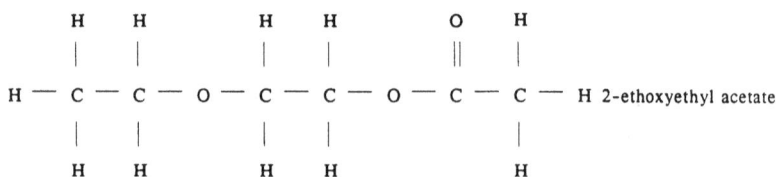

```
        H           H   H
        |           |   |
H ─── C ── O ── C ── C ── OH        2-methoxyethanol
        |           |   |
        H           H   H
```

```
        H   H           H   H
        |   |           |   |
H ─── C ── C ── O ── C ── C ── OH        2-ethoxyethanol
        |   |           |   |
        H   H           H   H
```

```
        H           H   H           O   H
        |           |   |           ||  |
H ─── C ── O ── C ── C ── O ── C ── C ── H        2-methoxyethyl acetate
        |           |   |               |
        H           H   H               H
```

```
        H   H           H   H           O   H
        |   |           |   |           ||  |
H ─── C ── C ── O ── C ── C ── O ── C ── C ── H  2-ethoxyethyl acetate
        |   |           |   |               |
        H   H           H   H               H
```

Information on the identity of the four selected glycol ethers is presented in Table 1.

2.2 Physical and Chemical Properties

A summary of the physical and chemical properties of these four glycol ethers (2-ME; 2-MEA; 2-EE; 2-EEA) is given in Table 2.

2.3 Conversion Factors

2-Methoxyethanol (2-ME)	1 ppm = 3.11 mg/m^3
2-Methoxyethyl Acetate (2-MEA)	1 ppm = 4.83 mg/m^3
2-Ethoxyethanol (2-EE)	1 ppm = 3.68 mg/m^3
2-Ethoxyethyl Acetate (2-EEA)	1 ppm = 5.40 mg/m^3

2.4 Analytical Methods

Several analytical procedures used for the determination of 2-ME, 2-MEA, 2-EE, and 2-EEA in various environmental media are summarized in Table 3. In some reports, the useful range was indicated but not the limit of detection.

In reporting the methods validated by NIOSH (1987a, 1987b), only the range that has been confirmed as accurate is shown. However, these methods may be capable of measuring much lower levels of glycol ethers in air providing adequate sampling times are employed and desorption efficiencies ascertained.

Variations on the basic NIOSH sampling and gas chromatographic methods have been reported by Denkhaus et al. (1986), and the measurement of glycol ethers in the workplace using diffusive monitors has been described by Hamlin et al. (1982).

Metabolites of 2-EE and 2-ME in urine have been measured using either gas chromatography (Groeseneken et al., 1986a, 1989b; Smallwood et al., 1984, 1988), or HPLC analysis (Cheever et al., 1984).

Using methylene chloride extractions of acidified urine, followed by derivatization with pentafluorobenzyl bromide, average recoveries of 78 and 91% were obtained for methoxyacetic acid (MAA) and ethoxyacetic acid (EAA),

Table 1. The identity of selected glycol ethers

Chemical	CAS Number	Molecular formula	Common synonyms	Some common trade names
2-Methoxyethanol (2-ME)	109-86-4	$C_3H_8O_2$	Ethylene glycol monomethyl ether; ethanol, 2-methoxy; EGM ether	Methyl Cellosolve; Jeffersol EM; Dowanol EM; Poly-solv EM; Methyl oxitol.
2-Methoxyethyl acetate (2-MEA)	110-49-6	$C_5H_{10}O_3$	Ethylene glycol monomethyl ether acetate; ethanol, 2-methoxy-acetate	Methyl Cellosolve acetate
2-Ethoxyethanol (2-EE)	110-80-5	$C_4H_{10}O_2$	Ethylene glycol monoethyl ether	Cellosolve, Dowanol EE; Oxitol; Ethoxol
2-Ethoxyethyl acetate (2-EEA)	111-15-9	$C_6H_{12}O_3$	Ethylene glycol monoethyl ether acetate; acetic acid, 2-ethoxyethyl ester.	Cellosolve acetate; Ethyl Cellosolve acetate; Oxitol acetate; Poly-Solv EE

Table 2. Physical and chemical properties of selected glycol ethers[a]

Chemical	Relative molecular mass	Density (g/ml at 20 °C)	Boiling point (°C)	Vapour pressure (mmHg)	Relative vapour density (air = 1)	Flash point (°C)	Water solubility
2-Methoxyethanol (2-ME)	76.09	0.960	124	6.2 at 20 °C 9.7 at 25 °C	2.6	46.1 open cup 41.7 closed cup	Infinite
2-Methoxyethyl Acetate (2-MEA)	118.13	1.005	145	2.0 at 20 °C 5.3 at 25 °C	4.07	55.6 closed cup	Infinite
2-Ethoxyethanol (2-EE)	90.12	0.93	135	3.8 at 20 °C 5.3 at 25 °C	3.0	49 open cup 44 closed cup	Infinite
2-Ethoxyethyl Acetate (2-EEA)	132.16	0.975	156	1.2 at 20 °C 1.1 at 25 °C	4.72	51.1 closed cup	23 g/100g at 20 °C

[a] Data from: Rowe & Wolf (1982) and Mellan (1977)

respectively. Detection limits for GC-FID analysis were 11.4 µg/ml for MAA and 5.0 µg/ml for EAA (Smallwood et al., 1984). Smallwood et al. (1988) have reported that a range of 5 to 100 µg EAA/ml in urine can be analysed. Preliminary results indicate that this procedure can be used to detect exposure to 2-EE in shipyard workers using 2-EE-containing paints. Groeseneken et al. (1986a) utilized similar extraction procedures and GC-FID analysis after diazomethane derivatization. Although recoveries were low (50-60%), the method could quantify 0.15 mg MAA per litre and 0.07 mg EAA/litre. Groeseneken et al. (1989b) have recently described an improved method for detecting MAA and EAA in urine. Recoveries were in excess of 90%, linear standard curves were obtained over a broad range (0.1-200 mg/litre), and the possible interference by gly-colic acid in the assay previously described (Groeseneken et al. 1986a) was eliminated. Cheever et al. (1984) ana-lysed urine samples, directly at pH 3 by HPLC, for EAA after animals were dosed with 230 mg 2-EE/kg body weight, but no limit of detection or appropriate range for use was reported. However, this method may be useful for biological monitoring of exposed populations.

Table 3. Analytical methods for selected glycol ethers and their metabolites

Matrix	Sampling method extraction/cleanup	Analytical method[a]	Limit of detection or useful range	Reference
Air	Adsorption on charcoal, elution with methylene chloride, carbon disulfide or methylene chloride; methanol	GC-FID	range (mg/m^3): 2-ME 44-160; 2-MEA 51-214; 2-EE 340-1460	NIOSH (1987a, 1987b)
Air (2-EE)	Inhaled or expired air pumped through silica gel, desorbed with methanol (88% efficient)	GC-FID	NR	Groeseneken et al. (1986b)
Air (2-ME, 2-EE)	Diffusive sampling, adsorption on Tenax thermal desorption	GC-FID	range: 5-20 mg/m^3	Hamlin et al. (1982)
Air (2-ME, 2-EE)	Personal monitors with pump adsorption on Tenax thermal desorption	GC-FID	range: 0.5-250 mg/m^3	Health and Safety Executive (1988)
Water (2-EEA)	Direct analysis of aqueous solutions	HPLC-UV	5 mg/litre; range: 5-1000 mg/litre	Bailey et al. (1985)

Table 3 (contd)

Matrix	Sampling method extraction/cleanup	Analytical method[a]	Limit of detection or useful range	Reference
Blood (2-ME, 2-EE)	Methylene chloride extraction in presence of anhydrous sodium sulfate. Average recoveries 2-ME (78%), 2-EE (84%)	GC-FID	2-ME 8.8 mg/kg; range 8-946 mg/kg 2-EE 5.0 mg/kg; range 6-895 mg/kg	Smallwood et al. (1984)
Blood (2-ME, 2-EE)	Head-space elution	GC-FID	NR	Denkhaus et al. (1986)
Urine (MAA, EAA)	Methylene extraction followed by derivatization with pentafluorobenzyl bromide	GC-FID	MAA 11.4 mg/litre; range 11.4-1140 mg/litre EAA 5.0 mg/litre; range 10-1000 mg/litre	Smallwood et al. (1984)
Urine (MAA, EAA)	Lyophilization followed by derivatization with pentafluorobenzyl	GC-FID	MAA 0.03 mg/litre; range 0.1-200 mg/litre EAA 0.03 mg/litre; range 0.1-200 mg/litre	Groeseneken et al. (1989b)

[a] GC-FID = gas chromatography-flame ionization detector; HPLC-UV = high performance liquid chromatography with ultraviolet light detection; NR = not reported.

3. SOURCES OF HUMAN AND ENVIRONMENTAL EXPOSURE

3.1 Natural Occurrence

The two glycol ethers and their acetates (2-ME, 2-MEA, 2-EE, 2-EEA) have not been reported to occur as natural products.

3.2 Man-Made Sources

3.2.1 Industrial production

3.2.1.1 Manufacturing processes

The production process for 2-ME and 2-EE involves the reaction of the relevant alcohol with ethylene oxide to produce the required glycol ether (Kirk-Othmer, 1980). The acetates, 2-MEA and 2-EEA, are produced by standard esterification techniques using 2-ME or 2-EE, the acid anhydride or chloride, and an acid catalyst (Kirk-Othmer, 1980).

3.2.1.2 World production figures

The use of 2-ME and 2-EE has declined over the past few years because they have been partially replaced in some countries by less toxic substances. Estimates of production levels for three major industrialized areas are shown in Table 4. Production figures for other regions of the world have not been found.

Table 4. Estimated production (in tonnes) of 2-EE and 2-ME in 1981[a]

Region or Country	2-ME	2-EE
Western Europe	37 000	116 000
Japan	3100	9800
United States	39 000	79 000

[a] These are estimates taken from US EPA (1987); production figures for the rest of the world have not been found.

3.3   Uses

2-ME, 2-EE, 2-MEA, and 2-EEA have a wide range of uses as solvents with particular applications in paints, stains, inks, lacquers, and the production of food-contact plastics. The major function of these agents is to dissolve various components of mixtures, in both aqueous and non-aqueous systems, and to keep them in solution until the last stages of evaporation. It is these dispersive applications that cause the greatest concern for widespread human and environmental exposure.

In addition, these four glycol ethers are used as resin solvents, in surface coatings and inks for silk-screen printing and in photographic and photolithographic processes, as solvents for dyes in textile and leather finishing, and as general solvents in a wide variety of home and industrial cleaners. 2-ME is used extensively as an anti-icing additive in hydraulic fluids and jet fuel for military and small civilian jet aircraft, as well as in hydraulic brake fluids (Mellan, 1977).

4. ENVIRONMENTAL TRANSPORT, DISTRIBUTION, AND TRANSFORMATION

4.1 Transport and Distribution Between Media

The greatest environmental exposure to glycol ethers results from their direct release into the atmosphere when they are used as evaporative solvents. Given the amounts synthesized and transported, there is also a great potential for environmental exposure from accidental releases and the disposal of cleaning products and containers. Discharges of this type result in the transport of these chemicals to land and water. Because of their water solubility and low vapour pressure, they could build up in water in the absence of degradation. However, their levels in soil and water would be expected to decrease fairly quickly because of rapid hydrolysis and/or oxidation. Also, adapted sludge has been reported to digest these compounds (Verschueren, 1977), giving 90% degradation of 2-EE after 5.5 days.

Since all of the major degradation processes in soil and water are oxidative, the potential exists for persistent contamination of anaerobic soils, such as landfills, and their underlying anaerobic aquifers. Contamination of ground water by 2-EE and 2-EEA from leaking storage tanks has been observed (Botta et al., 1984). However, 2-ME can apparently serve as a substrate for anaerobic methane fermentation and is digested by anaerobic sludge (Tanaka et al., 1986). Under such conditions, contamination of soil and ground water would be transitory.

4.2 Biotransformation

Under normal aerobic conditions, 2-ME, 2-EE, and their acetates would be expected to be degraded readily to carbon dioxide and water by microorganisms. Under anaerobic conditions, 2-ME is degraded by mesophilic sludge through at least two pathways, depending on temperature and pH, with methane and carbon dioxide being the end products in both cases (Tanaka et al., 1986). Optimal conditions for degradation are pH 7.5 and 30-35°C.

5. ENVIRONMENTAL LEVELS AND HUMAN EXPOSURE

5.1 Environmental Levels

The patterns of use of these four glycol ethers can result in significant, widespread emissions to the environment. Therefore, there is a great potential for exposure to people in the workplace, as well as to the general population and to the environment. However, no data on the levels of 2-ME, 2-EE, and their acetates in the general environment have been found. As a result of the rates of degradation and the physical and chemical properties of these compounds, it is highly unlikely that food chain accumulation would occur.

5.2 General Population Exposure

No data have been found that would allow an estimate to be made of the exposure to the general population using these evaporative solvents. However, there is particular concern for direct human exposure in small workshops and by individual users, where the products are being used in environments with either poor or non-existent ventilation, or where skin exposure may not be controlled adequately.

5.3 Occupational Exposure

Workers, other than those in large industrial establishments, constitute the largest population group subject to high exposure. In the USA, airborne exposures have been measured for some of the trades, many of the industrial uses, and for workers involved in the manufacture of these compounds (Table 5). In a survey of European manufacturing sites, the time-weighted averages (TWAs) for workers exposed to 2-ME, 2-MEA, 2-EE, and 2-EEA were reported as 28.9, 4.3, 15.8, and 14.6 mg/m^3 (9.3, 0.9, 4.3, and 2.7 ppm), respectively (ECETOC, 1985). As estimates of exposure, these measurements do not take into account dermal or aerosol exposures, which may be very significant (see section 9.2). A summary of the exposure of workers in the semiconductor industry to 2-ME, 2-MEA, 2-EE, or 2-EEA

(Table 6) (Paustenbach, 1988) reports exposures lower than those in other industries within the USA (Table 5). These measurements do not accurately reflect exposure during uses such as maintenance painting (as opposed to industrial production), because here there is a wide variation in exposure conditions. Modelling of the possible range of exposures in trade and consumer uses might provide some useful data.

The exposure data available from large industries suggest that the majority of exposures are "low", i.e. exposures for 2-ME are below 0.1 mg/m^3 (0.03 ppm) and for 2-EE are below 1.8 mg/m^3 (0.5 ppm). However, in almost all industries studied there are some workers exposed to much higher levels (see section 9). For example, monitoring carried out in a number of industries using glycol ethers (Hamlin et al., 1982) involved both personal and area monitoring and covered a range of applications in flexographic and gravure printing, car refinishing, film coating, and printing ink manufacture. Although atmospheric concentrations were generally low, levels of up to 74 mg 2-EE/m^3 (20 ppm) and 146 mg 2-ME/m^3 (47 ppm) were reported in some poorly ventilated areas. There was wide variation in the exposure between different plants, even when these plants used the same process.

Air samples (2654 total) from 336 plants in Belgium have been analysed for glycol ethers (including 2-ME, 2-EE, and their acetates) (Veulemans et al., 1987b). One or more glycol ethers were detected in 262 air samples covering 78 plants, 2-EE and its acetate being detected most often. Detectable levels were of the order of 9.2 mg per m^3, 25% being above 18.4 mg/m^3.

Engineering models have been used to estimate exposure resulting from the use of paint, coatings, stains, etc., containing 2-ME, 2-EE, and their acetates. Such models indicate that peak exposure values of > 30 ppm and 1-h average exposures of > 5 ppm will occur when paints and similar products containing more than 2% of these solvents are used (US EPA, 1987). Much higher exposure levels are possible when the concentration of 2-ME or 2-EE in the paint is higher. These estimates apply to situations where protective equipment or special engineering controls were not available. Under industrial conditions, exposure may be lower than these models predict if ventilation, exhaust hoods, or other protective equipment are used.

Table 5. Summary of occupational exposures (mg/m³) to glycol ethers in the USA[a]

Chemical and job category	Arithmetic range[b]		Arithmetic mean	Standard deviation	Geometric mean	Geometric deviation
2-ME[c]						
Operator	0.31-188.5	(0.1 -60.6)	59.28 (19.06)	8.40 (2.70)	23.10 (7.43)	56.98 (18.32)
Miscellaneous			9.33 (3.00)	3.11 (1.00)	9.33 (3.00)	
Painter	0.31- 10.3	(0.1 - 3.3)	6.87 (2.21)	7.43 (2.39)	2.08 (0.67)	7.43 (2.39)
Painter/screener	0.31- 12.1	(0.1 - 3.9)	6.22 (2.00)	7.15 (2.30)	1.95 (0.63)	5.91 (1.90)
2-ME[d]						
Painter	3.76- 18.7	(1.21- 6.01)	11.23 (3.61)	5.69 (1.83)	8.40 (2.70)	7.46 (2.40)
Operator	5.19- 7.68	(1.67- 2.47)	6.44 (2.07)	3.76 (1.21)	6.31 (2.03)	1.24 (0.40)
2-ME[e]						
Operator	0.31- 35.14	(0.1 -11.3)	7.28 (2.34)	9.39 (3.02)	1.37 (0.44)	11.26 (3.62)
2-MEA[c]						
Miscellaneous	0.48- 40.57	(0.1 - 8.4)	12.94 (2.68)	13.09 (2.71)	1.69 (0.35)	16.81 (3.48)
Operator	0.48- 26.56	(0.1 - 5.5)	7.87 (1.63)	13.04 (2.70)	1.98 (0.41)	10.19 (2.11)
Printer/screener	0.48- 5.07	(0.1 - 1.05)	2.13 (0.44)	16.23 (3.36)	0.87 (0.18)	3.86 (0.80)
Painter	0.48- 14.49	(0.1 - 3.0)	1.88 (0.39)	15.94 (3.30)	0.77 (0.16)	3.31 (0.70)
2-EE[c]						
Painting	0.37-313.9	(0.1 -85.3)	71.21 (19.35)	13.69 (3.72)	2.72 (0.74)	74.30 (20.19)
Printer	0.37- 87.95	(0.1 -23.9)	17.77 (4.83)	9.09 (2.47)	4.49 (1.22)	19.95 (5.42)
Coating/adhesive	0.37-36.80	(0.1 -10.0)	5.89 (1.60)	13.14 (3.57)	0.99 (0.27)	11.85 (3.22)
Mechanical industry				0.37 (0.10)	3.68 (1.00)	0.04 (0.01)
Leather			0.37 (0.10)	3.68 (1.00)	0.04 (0.01)	
Operation/prod.			0.37 (0.10)	3.68 (1.00)	0.04 (0.01)	

3

Table 5 (contd).

Chemical and Job category	Arithmetic range[b]		Arithmetic mean	Standard deviation	Geometric mean	Geometric deviation
2-EE[d]						
Printer/screener	6.92-161.9	(1.88-44.0)	84.90 (23.07)	6.92 (1.88)	59.80 (16.25)	59.28 (16.11)
Operator	0.37- 9.86	(0.1-2.82)	0.66 (0.18)	10.38 (2.82)	0.15 (0.04)	0.92 (0.25)
2-EE[e]						
Printer/screener	0.37- 54.10	(0.1-14.79)	16.74 (4.55)	9.02 (2.45)	3.35 (0.91)	18.58 (5.05)
Miscellaneous			0.37 (0.10)	3.68 (1.00)	0.37 (0.10)	
2-EEA[c]						
Leather	6.75- 51.30	(1.25-9.5)	30.89 (5.72)	9.34 (1.73)	22.90 (4.24)	18.36 (3.40)
Paint, varnish, & coating	0.54-272.38	(0.1-50.44)	20.79 (3.85)	21.98 (4.07)	2.70 (0.50)	51.68 (9.57)
Printer	0.54- 53.46	(0.1- 9.9)	16.59 (3.07)	12.15 (2.25)	5.02 (0.93)	16.04 (2.97)
Prod./maint.	0.54- 27.0	(0.1- 5.0)	9.50 (1.76)	13.77 (2.55)	2.59 (0.48)	11.29 (2.09)
2-EEA[d]						
Painter	1.03- 5.08	(0.19-0.94)	3.08 (0.57)	9.88 (1.83)	2.27 (0.42)	2.05 (0.38)
Operator	3.56- 12.96	(0.66-2.4)	2.54 (0.47)	14.90 (2.76)	1.46 (0.27)	3.40 (0.63)
2-EA[e]						
Miscellaneous	15.12-230.04	(2.8-42.6)	67.61 (12.52)	14.04 (2.60)	36.72 (6.80)	82.57 (15.29)

[a] From: US EPA (1987). Values were reported as ppm in the original report and are given in parentheses.
[b] Values of 0.1 ppm or less are reported as 0.1 ppm.
[c] Federal (USA) OSHA data.
[d] California OSHA data.
[e] NIOSH data.

Table 6. Exposure to glycol ethers within the semiconductor industry in the USA (mg/m³)[a]

Sampling data	No.	2-EEA Range	2-EEA Mean + SD	No.	2-ME Range	2-ME Mean + SD	No.	2-MEA Range	2-MEA Mean + SD
Personal (TWA)	96	0.0054-2.7	0.27±0.43	6	0.12 -3.11	0.68±1.18	16	ND	0.048±0.00
Personal (Short-term)	21	0.0054-97.2	15.23±29.2	1	NA	80.0	1	NA	82.0
Area (TWA)	128	0.0054-9.72	0.27±0.86	4	0.093-2.49	0.72±1.18	20	ND	0.048±0.00
Area (Short-term)	10	0.027-81.0	8.42±25.49	1	NA	80.9	1	NA	87.0

[a] From: Paustenbach (1988).
No. = number of samples.
Analytical limit of detection: 2-EEA, 0.0054 mg/m³; 2-ME, 0.093 mg/³; and 2-MEA, 0.048 mg/m³.
TWA = time-weighted average.
NA = not applicable.
ND = not detectable.
SD = standard deviation.

6. KINETICS AND METABOLISM

6.1   Absorption

As would be expected from their chemical structures and solubilities, all four glycol ethers are readily absorbed through the skin, lungs, and gastrointestinal tract. Utilizing *in vitro* techniques, a rate of absorption of 2-EEA through beagle skin of 2.3 mg/cm^2 per h has been measured (Guest et al., 1984). For isolated human epidermis, the following absorption rates have been determined: 2-ME, 2.8 mg/cm^2 per h; 2-EE, 0.8 mg/cm^2 per h; and 2-EEA, 0.8 mg per cm^2 per h (Dugard et al., 1984).

In vivo studies in humans showed rapid absorption of 2-ME after dermal application of 15 ml of solvent (Nakaaki et al., 1980). Two hours after application, blood levels reached 200-300 μg/ml. This rate of absorption was approximately 10 times greater than that of methanol, acetone, or methyl acetate.

Indirect evidence exists to show that 2-EE is well absorbed from the gastrointestinal tract of rats. After a single oral dose of ^{14}C-2EE (230 mg/kg body weight), 76-80% of the dose was excreted in the urine within 96 h (Cheever et al., 1984).

6.2   Distribution

Glycol ethers are rapidly metabolized and eliminated in the mammalian species that have been studied (see sections 6.3 and 6.4). Very few studies have therefore been conducted to examine tissue distribution.

Using radioactive 2-ME, Sleet et al. (1986) noted that radioactivity was present throughout the maternal and conceptus compartments only 5 min after oral administration of a tracer dose to pregnant mice. The highest levels were noted in maternal liver, blood, and gastrointestinal tract, and in the placenta, yolk sac, and embryonic structures such as limb buds, somites, and neuroepithelium. Maternal blood levels declined to between 2 and 10% of peak levels after 24 h. At 6 h post-administration, 69% of the radioactivity in maternal liver and 33% of that in the embryo were acid soluble.

6.3 Metabolic Transformation

The glycol ether acetates, 2-EEA and 2-MEA, are rapidly hydrolysed *in vivo* to the free glycol ether (2-EE and 2-ME, respectively) and acetate in rats (Romer et al., 1985). The metabolism of 2-ME has been studied by Miller et al. (1983a) and Moss et al. (1985), who found that methoxyacetic acid (MAA) and methoxyacetyl glycine are the primary metabolites. MAA accounted for 50 to 60% of the urinary radioactivity and methoxyacetyl glycine for 18 to 25% during the 48-h observation period following a single intraperitoneal dose of 2-[methoxy-^{14}C]ethanol (250 mg per kg body weight) (Moss et al., 1985). The conversion in plasma of 2-ME to 2-MAA was rapid, the half-life for the disappearance of 2-ME being 36 min. In the study reported by Miller et al. (1983a) using ^{14}C labelled 2-ME, 12% of the dose was eliminated as $^{14}CO_2$ after 48 h, suggesting that either 2-ME or its metabolite 2-MAA underwent further oxidative metabolism.

2-Ethoxyacetic acid (EAA) and 2-ethoxyacetyl glycine have been found in the urine of rats that had been administered a single oral dose of 230 mg 2-EE/kg body weight (Cheever et al., 1984).

Fig. 1 shows the proposed pathway for the metabolism of 2-ME in the rat (Miller et al., 1983a; Moss et al., 1985; Foster et al., 1986). This route of metabolism involves the enzyme alcohol dehydrogenase (ADH), as shown by the blocking of 2-ME metabolism by the known ADH inhibitor 4-methylpyrazole (Moss et al., 1985). In addition, the administration of ethanol before exposure of rats to 2-ME or 2-EE has been found to prolong the retention of these glycol ethers in the blood (Romer et al., 1985). This effect was noted at ethanol blood levels above 3 mmole/litre. The retention of 2-ME or 2-EE in the body was attributed to the competitive inhibition by ethanol of the common metabolizing enzyme, alcohol dehydrogenase.

When rats were administered 2-EE at doses from 0.5 mg/kg to 100 mg/kg, Groeseneken et al. (1988) found increasing relative amounts of EAA in urine (from 13.4% to 36.8% of the total dose). This could be the result of competition by other metabolic pathways, which would become more easily saturated at the higher dosage levels.

$$CH_3 \; - \; O \; - \; CH_2 \; - \; CH_2 \; - \; OH$$

2-methoxyethanol

alcohol dehydrogenase $\quad \downarrow$ NADH

$$CH_3 \; - \; O \; - \; CH_2 \; - \; \overset{\displaystyle O}{\overset{\displaystyle \|}{C}} \; - \; H$$

methoxyacetaldehyde

aldehyde dehydrogenase $\quad \downarrow$ NADH

$$CH_3 \; - \; O \; - \; CH_2 \; - \; \overset{\displaystyle O}{\overset{\displaystyle \|}{C}} \; - \; OH$$

methoxyacetic acid

$$\downarrow$$

$$CH_3 \; - \; O \; - \; CH_2 \; - \; \overset{\displaystyle O}{\overset{\displaystyle \|}{C}} \; - \; NHCH_2COOH$$

Glycine conjugate

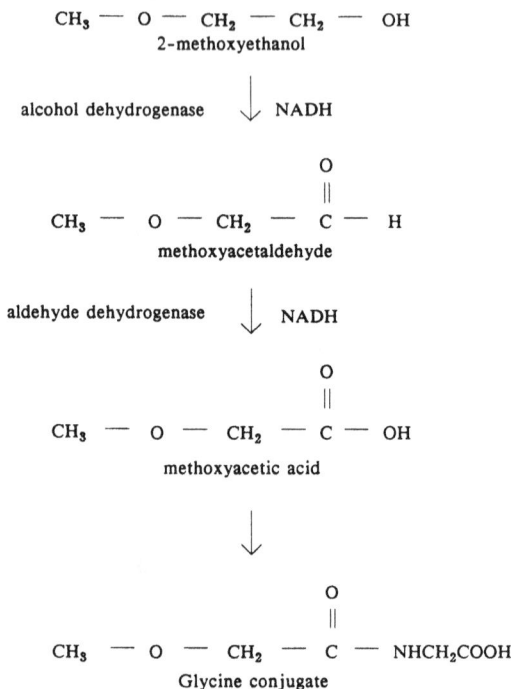

Fig. 1 Major metabolic pathway of 2-methoxyethanol in rats.

At 2-EE doses equivalent to the lowest doses in these animal studies, it was estimated that humans excrete 30-35% as EAA. Furthermore, 27% (on average) of the EAA was excreted as the glycine conjugate in the rat, whereas no glycine conjugation was observed in humans.

The *in vitro* nasal mucosal carboxylesterase activity of mice was compared to the activity of other mice tissues and to the nasal mucosal carboxylesterase activity of rats, rabbits, or dogs when exposed to 2-MEA or 2-EEA (Stott & McKenna, 1985). The specific activity in nasal carboxylase was found to be similar to that of the liver in mice, but it was greater than the activity found in the kidney, lung, or blood of mice. Nasal mucosal carboxylesterase activity of mice was comparable to that of dogs, slightly higher than the activity in rats, and nearly six-fold higher than the activity in rabbits. These *in vitro* studies suggest that considerable hydrolysis may occur in the intact animal, resulting in the formation of acetic acid at the initial route of entry.

6.4   Elimination and Excretion

Although 2-ME is rapidly metabolized to 2-MAA after an intraperitoneal dose of 250 mg/kg body weight in the rat, the excretion of 2-MAA is fairly slow (half-life of approximately 20 h) (Moss et al., 1985). In humans, an elimination half-life for 2-MAA of 77.1 h has been reported (Groeseneken et al., 1989a). The elimination of radioactive 2-EAA (ethyl 1,2^{14}C) has been reported in the rat (half-life of approximately 8 h) (Guest et al., 1984) and in humans (half-life of approximately 21-42 h) (Groeseneken, 1986b,c, 1988; Veulemans, 1987a). In rats, the administration of an oral dose of 230 mg 2-EE/kg body weight led to the production of EAA and N-ethoxyacety glycine (> 76% of the dose), EAA being the major metabolite found in testes after 2 h (Cheever et al., 1984).

The urinary excretion of EAA during and after single 4-h exposures to 14, 28, or 50 mg 2-EEA/m^3 in human volunteers has been reported by Groeseneken et al. (1987). The distribution/excretion time course during and after 2-EEA exposure was similar to that observed for 2-EE. This indicates that humans, like rodents, hydrolyse the acetate to 2-EE, which is then converted to the EAA metabolite and excreted. The excretion of the EAA metabolite was observed to be biphasic. A second peak of excretion occurred approximately 3 h after the first, suggesting some type of redistribution of the glycol ethers, or of a metabolite, from a peripheral compartment.

The urinary excretion of EAA was evaluated under field conditions in which women volunteers were exposed daily to 2-EE or 2-EEA in the process of silk-screen printing (Veulemans et al., 1987a). Urinary EAA was measured during 5 days of normal production and was also detectable after a 12-day stop in production. The excretion of EAA increased during the work week, yet it was still detectable after 12 days without exposure. These data suggest that the retention of EAA, or of other 2-EE or 2-EEA metabolite, may be toxicologically significant if EAA is the active metabolite responsible for the observed toxicity.

7. EFFECTS ON ORGANISMS IN THE ENVIRONMENT

Given the physical and chemical properties of these four glycol ethers and the known rates of degradation in the environment (section 4), there is minimal concern that hazardous levels of these substances will occur. Although only a few studies have been reported, the available data support this conclusion. For example, both 2-ME and 2-EE have been tested for effects on microorganisms and aquatic animals. The lethal concentration of 2-ME and 2-EE to microorganisms (*Cladosporium resinae, Pseudomonas aeruginosa, Gliomastix* sp, and *Candida* sp is > 2% in the medium (Neihof & Bailey, 1978; Lee & Wong, 1979). The exposure of *C. resinae* lasted 30 to 42 days, whereas the other organisms were exposed for 4 months. Very low toxicity was shown by 2-ME to the green alga *Scenedesmus quadricauda* (growth inhibition only at > 10 g/litre) and the cyano-bacterium (blue-green alga) *Microcystis aeruginosa* (growth inhibition only at > 100 mg/litre) (Bringmann & Kuhn, 1978). 2-EE has very low toxicity to the brine shrimp *(Artemia salina)* (LC_{50} > 4 g/litre) (Price et al., 1974) and to another arthropod *Daphnia magna* (Hermens et al., 1984). The toxicity of 2-EE to freshwater fish is also very low, the LC_{50} (96 h) for the bluegill *(Lepomis macrochirus)* being > 10 g/litre. However, 2-EEA is far more toxic to fish in this assay, LC_{50} (96 h) values of 60 mg/litre (Bailey et al., 1985) and 46 mg per litre in fathead minnows *(Pimephales promelas)* (Purdy, 1987) having been reported. These results confirm those of Juhnke & Ludemann (1978), who reported an LC_{50} (48 h) value of 107-141 mg per litre when using the Golden Orfe *(Leuciscus idus melanotus)* test. The reason for this low LC_{50} has not been studied, but Dawson et al. (1977) reported similarly low LC_{50} values for 2-MEA in fish (45 mg per litre in tidewater silverfish *(Menidia beryllina)* and bluegill *(Lepomis chirus)*.

Effects on other organisms have not been reported.

8. EFFECTS ON EXPERIMENTAL ANIMALS AND *IN VITRO* TEST SYSTEMS

8.1 Single Exposures

Data indicating the acute oral, dermal, intraperitoneal, and inhalation toxicities of 2-ME and 2-EE are given in Table 7. As shown, these two glycol ethers have similar toxicities, and are of low acute toxicity whether animals are exposed via the dermal, oral, or respiratory routes. Even after intraperitoneal injection, the reported levels of acute toxicity are still low (1.7-2.46 g per kg body weight).

Dyspnoea, somnolence, ataxia, and prostration were reported after near lethal doses of 2-EE were given to rats, mice, guinea-pigs, or rabbits (Stenger et al., 1971). Haemoglobinuria and/or haematuria were reported after a single oral administration of 2-EE with a dose approaching the LD_{50} (Laug et al., 1939). Microscopic examination of the kidneys of rats, mice, guinea-pigs, or rabbits given 2-EE orally revealed severe tubular degeneration, congestion, and cast formation; in some animals most of the cortical tubules were necrotic (Laug et al., 1939). No data on the purity of the 2-EE used in these early studies were reported.

Single 4-h inhalation exposures of rats to 1866 mg 2-ME per m^3 or more led to testicular atrophy as early as 24 h after exposure (Doe, 1984b).

8.2 Short-term Exposures

Repeated exposure of experimental animals to 2-ME and 2-EE by various routes of administration (7-90 days) have revealed adverse effects on the haematological and nervous systems and on the testes, thymus, kidney, liver, and lung. From data on the metabolic transformation and elimination of 2-MEA and 2-EEA in animals and man (see section 6), it is probable that the toxicities of these glycol ether acetates are similar to those of the parent chemicals 2-ME and 2-EE.

Table 7. Acute toxicity data for 2-methoxyethanol and 2-ethoxyethanol and their acetates[a]

Compound	Species	Intraperitoneal LD$_{50}$	Oral LD$_{50}$	Dermal LD$_{50}$	Inhalation LC$_{50}$	References
2-Methoxyethanol	Rat	2460	2460-3400			Smyth et al. (1941); Goldberg et al. (1962); Pisko & Verbilov (1988)
	Mouse	2200	2167-2560		4603 (1480)	Werner et al. (1943); Saparmamedov (1974); Pisko & Verbilov (1988) Karel et al. (1947)
	Guinea-pig		950			Carpenter et al. (1956); Pisko & Verbilov (1988)
	Rabbit		890-1450	1300		
2-Ethoxyethanol	Rat	2000	2125-5500			Smyth et al. (1941); Laug et al. (1939) Stenger et al. (1971); Pisko & Verbilov (1988)
	Mouse	1700	4000-4800		6698 (1820)	Werner et al. (1943); Laug et al (1939) Stenger et al. (1971); Saparmemedov (1974); Pisko & Verbilov (1988) Karel et al. (1947); Laug et al. (1939) Stenger et al. (1971); Smyth et al. (1941)
	Guinea-pig		1400-2600			
	Rabbit			3300-15 200		
2-Methoxyethanol acetate	Rat		3930			Smyth et al. (1941) Kirk-Othmer (1980)
	Guinea-pig		1250			
	Rabbit			5557		
2-Ethoxyethanol acetate	Rat		5100			Smyth et al. (1941) Kirk-Othmer (1980)
	Guinea-pig		1910			
	Rabbit			10 333		

[a] Doses are given as mg/kg body weight except for inhalation doses, which are in mg/m^3 (values in parentheses are ppm)

8.2.1 Haematological and immunological effects

Following repeated exposures to 2-ME and 2-EE using various routes of administration, haematological effects have been observed in several species. A summary of the most relevant studies is given in Tables 8 (2-ME) and 9 (2-EE).

Concerning changes in blood parameters, a comparison of Tables 7, 8, and 9 indicates clearly that 2-ME is more toxic than 2-EE in several species, although 2-EE has been less widely studied. For example, Nagano et al. (1979) showed that 2-EE administered orally for 5 weeks at 2000 mg/kg body weight per day did not result in changes in haematological parameters other than a reduced leucocyte count. No effects were observed at 1000 mg/kg. Under a similar dosing regimen, 2-ME caused a dose-related reduction in leucocytes at 500 mg/kg per day, other haematological parameters being unaffected at 250 mg/kg per day (Nagano et al., 1979).

Some of the doses used in the studies summarized in Tables 7 and 8 resulted in histological and functional changes in the bone marrow and thymus. In an inhalation study, Miller et al. (1983b) noted thymic atrophy and decreased thymus weights in male and female rats exposed to 933 mg 2-ME/m^3 for 13 weeks. Miller et al. (1981) also noted decreased weights of thymus, spleen, and mesenteric lymph nodes in rats exposed to 933 or 3110 mg 2-ME/m^3 for 9 days, and reduced bone marrow cellularity was observed at 3110 mg/m^3. In one study there was at least partial reversal of these effects 22 days after an exposure lasting 4 days (Grant et al., 1985).

When MAA, the metabolite of 2-ME, was administered to rats by gavage at 300 mg/kg body weight per day for 8 days, it resulted in reduced erythrocyte counts, haemoglobin concentrations, and packed cell volumes, and a marked reduction in leucocyte counts. Thymus and spleen weights were also decreased and a severe lymphoid depletion was seen in the thymus. Similar, but less marked, effects on blood and thymus were seen in some animals administered 100 mg/kg per day. No treatment-related effects were reported at 30 mg/kg per day (Miller et al., 1982).

Table 8. Haematological effects of 2-methoxyethanol in animals[a]

Species	Route	No.	Dose frequency; time; level	Effect	References
Rat	inhalation	10 males 10 females	6 h/day; 9 days; 311, 933, 3110 mg/m^3	RBC fragility, no effect at 3110 mg/m^3 but reduced RBC, Hb, and PCV levels and bone marrow cellularity seen in M and F; similar findings in F at 933 mg/m^3; reduced WBC at 3110 and 933 mg/m^3; reduced thymus weight	Miller et al. (1981)
Rat	inhalation	10 males 10 females	6 h/day; 5 days/week for 13 weeks; 93.3, 311, 933 mg/m^3	only effect at 2 lowest doses was reduced body weight gain in F; at 933 mg/m^3 reduced WBC, Hb, PCV, and platelets in both sexes after 4 and 12 weeks; reduced serum proteins at 13 weeks, thymic atrophy	Miller et al. (1983b)
Rabbit	inhalation	5 males 5 females	6 h/day; 5 days/week for 13 weeks; 93.3, 311, 933 mg/m^3	decreased thymus size and body weight, PCV, WBC, platelets and Hb at 933 mg/m^3; slight to moderate decrease in lymphoid tissue at 311 mg/m^3	Miller et al. (1983b)
Dog	inhalation	2 treated 2 controls	7 h/day; 5 days/week for 12 weeks; 750 mg/m^3	decreased RBC, Hb and Hct; increased immature granulocytes	Werner et al. (1943)

Table 8 (contd).

Species	Route	No.	Dose frequency; time; level	Effect	References
Mouse	oral	5 males	5 times/week for 5 weeks; 62.5, 125, 250, 500, 1000, 2000 mg/kg body weight/day	4/5 mice at 2000 mg/kg died before completion; doses at or above 500 mg/kg resulted in reduced WBC, RBC, and PCV	Nagano et al. (1979)
Rat	oral	24 males	once per day for 4 days; 100 and 500 mg/kg body weight/day; sacrificed	reduced thymus and spleen weight at 500 mg/kg on days 1-8, recovery by day 22; reduced WBC at both 100 and 500 mg/kg, largely reversible by day 22	Grant et al. (1985)
Hamster	oral	4 males	once daily, 5 days/week for 5 weeks; 62.5, 125, 500 mg/kg body weight/day	decrease in WBC at 500 mg/kg the only effect on blood	Nagano et al. (1984)
Guinea-pig	oral	3 males	once daily, 5 days/week for 5 weeks; 250 and 500 mg/kg body weight/day	about 50% decrease in WBC at both doses	Nagano et al. (1984)

a M = male; F = female; PCV = packed cell volume; Hct = haematocrit; RBC = red blood cell count; WBC = white blood cell count; Hb = haemoglobin; No. = number of animals per group

Table 9. Haematological effects of 2-ethoxyethanol in animals[a]

Species	Route	Number animals per group	Dose frequency; time; level	Response	Reference
Rat	Inhalation	15 males 15 females	6 h/day; 5 days/week for 13 weeks; 92, 368, 1472 mg/m³	decreased leucocyte count in females at 1472 mg/m³, no other significant biological effect reported	Barbee et al. (1984)
Rabbit	Inhalation	10 males 10 females	6 h/day; 5 days/week for 13 weeks; 92, 368, 1472 mg/m³	decreased Hb, Hct, and RBC in both males and females only at 1472 mg/m³	Barbee et al. (1984)
Dog	Inhalation	2 treated 2 control	7 h/day; 5 days/week for 12 weeks; 3091 mg/m³	slight reduction in RBC, Hb, and PCV, microcytosis, hypochromia, and poly-chromatophilia were seen, marked increase in immature granulocytes	Werner er al. (1943)
Mouse	oral	5 males	5 times/week for 5 weeks; 62.5, 125, 250, 500, 3110, 2000 mg/kg body weight/day	lower WBC at 2000 mg/kg, but no effect on erythrocyte parameters	Nagano et al. (1979)

[a] PCV = packed cell volume; Hct = haematocrit; RBC = red blood cell count; WBC = white blood cell count; Hb = haemoglobin

Studies on immunological function show that 2-ME and 2-EE yield different results. De Delbarre et al. (1980) studied the effect of 2-ME and 2-EE on the humoral responsiveness to antigenic stimuli and on adjuvant arthritis in the rat. 2-ME had an inhibitory effect on adjuvant arthritis at doses greater than 18.6 mg/kg body weight per day administered subcutaneously, whereas 2-EE was not effective at doses up to 150 mg/kg. A dose of 150 mg 2-ME per kg per day delayed rejection of skin grafts and 75 mg 2-ME/kg per day (for 28 days) significantly depressed antibody production. Again, 2-EE had no effect on these parameters. House et al. (1985) administered 2-ME to mice by gavage (10 doses of 250, 500, or 1000 mg 2-ME/kg body weight per day for 2 weeks) and noted a 48% reduction in thymus weight at 500 and 1000 mg/kg. However, there was no significant alteration in immune function or host resistance. Similar findings were reported when the same dose levels of MAA, the major metabolite of 2-ME (section 6), were administered.

8.2.2   Effects on liver and kidney

Effects on the liver, such as reduced cytoplasmic density, disruption of lobular structure, elevated plasma fibrinogen, reduced serum proteins, and elevated liver weights, have been reported in certain studies in which rats, mice, or rabbits were exposed to 2-ME or 2-EE at levels in excess of 300 ppm (933 and 1104 mg/m^3, respectively), for periods of up to 13 weeks. Many of the effects observed were reversible, and no consistent pattern was noted among the various studies (Miller et al., 1981; 1983b; Stenger et al., 1971). Hepatic changes have been observed at inhalation exposures to 2-ME and 2-EE in excess of 300 ppm (933 and 1104 mg/m^3, respectively).

No pathological changes could be detected in the kidneys of rats exposed to approximately 933 mg 2-ME/m^3 for 6 or 7 h per day, 5 days a week, for 13 weeks (Miller et al., 1981, 1983b). In studies with 2-EE, no treatment-related pathology was reported after inhalation exposure of rats to 1362 mg/m^3 (370 ppm) for 5 weeks or dogs to 3091 mg/m^3 (840 ppm) for 12 weeks (Werner et al., 1943).

8.2.3   Behavioural and neurological effects

There have been few reports on the effects of 2-ME and 2-EE on the function of the nervous system in animals. Ataxia was reported after inhalation exposure of rats to 18.96 g 2-EE/m³ (5152 ppm) for 8h. After exposure of rats to levels of 2-ME between 1555 and 12 440 mg/m³, 4 h per day for up to 7 days, inhibition of an avoidance-escape conditioned response was observed without any alteration of motor function (Goldberg et al., 1962). The same authors reported also a significant inhibition of this response after 14 days exposure to 1210-4836 mg 2-ME per m³ (389-1555 ppm). After 3 weeks recovery, rats whose avoidance response had been inhibited on the 14th day showed a return to normal. Savolainen (1980) reported a partial loss of motor function in the hind limbs of rats after exposure to 1244 mg 2-ME/m³ (400 ppm) for 6 h/day, 5 days per week, for 2 weeks. This hindlimb paralysis coincided with the glial cell toxicity noted during the second week of exposure. Recovery was incomplete after 2 weeks post-exposure, the animals receiving the highest dose showing minor paresis.

8.3   Skin and Eye Irritation; Sensitization

No satisfactory data on the sensitization potential of 2-ME and 2-EE in animals, and only limited data on their irritant properties to eyes, have been reported. Weil & Scala (1971) found 2-ME to be an eye irritant. Lailler et al. (1975) reported that 0.1 ml of undiluted 2-ME led to corneal and conjunctival oedema and increased vascular leakage in the conjunctiva and aqueous humour. A 25% aqueous solution was much less active.

8.4   Long-term Exposures

No adequate long-term animal studies on 2-ME and 2-EE or their acetates have been reported to date.

8.5   Effects on Reproduction and Fetal Development

The effects of glycol ethers, particularly 2-ME, on animal reproduction, fertility, and teratogenicity have been extensively studied. Some of the early studies on reproduction have been reviewed by Hardin (1983). The many studies conducted in several countries and in several animal species are in general agreement on the nature of developmental and reproductive effects.

8.5.1   Effects on the male reproductive system

8.5.1.1   Oral exposure

The pathological changes observed in the testes of rats after the administration of 2-ME have been well characterized by Foster et al. (1983). The severe degenerative changes noted in the germinal epithelium of the seminiferous tubules of different laboratory animals were similar, irrespective of species or route of administration. Daily doses of 2-ME were administered orally to rats (50, 100, 250, or 500 mg/kg) for periods between 1 and 11 days, and 250, 500, or 1000 mg 2-EE/kg body weight per day was administered in a similar regimen (Foster et al., 1983; Creasy & Foster, 1984; Creasy et al., 1985). After 2-ME administration, testicular damage was observed 1 day post dosing with 100 mg/kg or more, the lesion being localized in the late primary spermatocytes. Continuous dosing with 2-ME resulted not only in progressive deletion of the primary spermatocytes but also in degenerative changes in secondary spermatocytes and dividing spermatids. Changes in sperm motility, morphology, and concentration were also reported. The cessation in maturation of early primary spermatocytes led to a depletion of the spermatid population, resulting in tubules containing only Sertoli cells, spermatogonia, and early primary spermatocytes. Decreased testicular weight was reported at 250 mg per kg or more. Although most of the effects seen after a 4-day treatment with 2-ME were reversible within 8 weeks, a small proportion of tubules showed incomplete recovery indicating a non-reversible, long-term effect. Similar findings were reported after 2-EE administration, but only after 11 days of dosing with 500 and 1000 mg/kg. No effects on the testes were observed following oral administration of 250 mg 2-EE/kg per day or 50 mg 2-ME/kg per day.

Subsequent work by Chapin et al. (1985a,b) supports the hypothesis that 2-ME administered to male rats at doses of 100 or 200 mg/kg daily for 5 days affects the spermatogonia. In these studies male rats were given doses of 0, 50, 100, or 200 mg/kg per day for 5 days, and recovery was investigated by evaluating the testicular damage in sacrificed animals at 8 subsequent weekly intervals or alternatively by investigating fertility through mating with two females per week for 8 weeks. Treatment with 100 or 200 mg/kg resulted in widespread testicular damage and cell death immediately after treatment, with only very mild effects being noted at 50 mg/kg (this was thus a marginal-effect level rather than a no-effect level). There was some evidence of recovery from testicular damage towards the end of the study period, but reduced fertility was still apparent weeks after the cessation of treatment with 200 mg/kg. Thus, the recovery was neither as complete nor as rapid as that noted by Foster et al. (1983).

The *in vivo* and *in vitro* effects of 2-ME and MAA exposures, respectively, were compared by evaluating effects using electron microscopy (Creasy et al., 1986). 2-ME caused cell death in the pachytene spermatocytes *in vivo*, as well as focal breakdown of the plasma membranes between spermatocytes and Sertoli cells. Similar, but less frequent, breaks were seen *in vitro* when mixed cultures of Sertoli and germ cells were treated with MAA.

Subsequent studies by Foster et al. (1987), in which the alkoxyacetic acids of 2-ME and 2-EE (MAA and EAA, respectively) were given orally in doses equimolar to the studies described earlier (Foster et al., 1983), yielded similar patterns of testicular degeneration and effects on spermatocyte development. The similarity of effects at equimolar concentrations between the two acetic acid derivatives and their respective glycol ethers suggests that these metabolites may either be the causative factors or at least play a role in the production of the observed degenerative effects.

The assessment of the effects of low doses of potential toxicants on sperm fertility and production is difficult because of the large amount of sperm usually produced by most test species and the large sperm reserves. Using an experimental design that required bi-daily matings of Long-Evans male rats, the effects of orally administered 2-EE (0, 150, or 300 mg/kg body weight per day; 5 days per week for 6 weeks) on sperm reserves and on pachytene spermatocytes was evaluated (Hurtt & Zenick, 1986). Further groups of rats received the same doses of 2-EE, but were not subjected to repeated mating. After 6 weeks of treatment, the animals were sacrificed and the effect of 2-EE administration on organ weight, testicular spermatid count, cauda epididymal sperm count, and sperm morphology was determined. Exposures to 2-EE resulted in significant decreases in testicular weight, spermatid count, and epididymal sperm count for both mated and unmated animals at the highest dose level. However, the effects were also seen at 150 mg/kg per day in repeatedly mated animals.

Adult male rats treated orally with 2-EE (936 mg/kg body weight, 5 days/week for 6 weeks) were found to have decreased sperm counts and altered sperm morphologies after 5 and 6 weeks of exposure when compared with vehicle-control animals, and sperm motility was decreased at week 6 (Oudiz & Zenick, 1986). These data indicate that the pachytene spermatocyte is the target cell most sensitive to the effects of 2-EE.

The reproductive toxicity of 2-EE in CD-1 mice has been evaluated in a continuous breeding protocol (Lamb et al., 1984). Male and female mice (20 males and 20 females per dose group) were given access to drinking-water containing 0.5, 1.0, or 2.0% 2-EE and housed as breeding pairs continuously for 14 weeks. Treated animals were then paired with controls for breeding. At 1 and 2% 2-EE, significant adverse effects on fertility were seen, the reproductive capacity of both males and females being affected. Testicular atrophy, decreased sperm motility, and increased abnormal sperm levels were seen in treated males, but no treatment-related pathological effects were seen in females even though reduced fertility was noted in the cross-mating phase.

The reproductive toxicity of a single oral dose of 2-ME (0, 500, 750, 1000, or 1500 mg/kg) was assessed in adult male CD rats and CD-1 mice by Anderson et al. (1987). Animals from each group were sacrificed at weekly intervals during weeks 3-8 post exposure and evaluated for sperm counts, sperm morphology, and testicular histology. A dose-related toxicological response in spermatocytes was observed in both species. In a companion study, male rats and mice were exposed to 2-ME (0, 125, 250, or 500 mg/kg) and permitted to mate during weeks 1-10 post exposure. Following mating, pregnant females were sacrificed on day 17 of pregnancy and each uterus was evaluated for dominant lethal effects. The only effect noted was a decrease in total number of implants at week 6 following treatment with 500 mg/kg. In a study in which both rats and mice were given single doses at 0, 500, 750, 1000, or 1500 mg per kg and mated 5 and 6 weeks later, dominant lethal studies showed a dose-related decrease in fertility in rats, with complete sterility in all but the lowest dose group after 6 weeks. No effects on the reproductive capacity of mice were noted. There was no statistically significant evidence for the induction of dominant lethal mutations or abnormalities in the F_1 generation of either species.

8.5.1.2 Inhalation studies

Testicular damage has been reported in rats exposed to 2-ME by inhalation for a single 4-h period (Doe, 1984b). Exposure to 1944 mg/m^3 resulted in histological evidence of damage to the maturing spermatids, testicular atrophy occurring at 3887 mg/m^3 or more. The NOEL was 933 mg/m^3.

The effect of *repeated* exposure to 2-ME has also been investigated using the inhalation route. Exposure of rats to 3110 mg/m^3 (6 h/day) for 9 out of 11 days resulted in degenerative changes and necrosis in the germinal epithelium of the seminiferous tubules, but no effects on the testes were observed with a dose of 933 mg/m^3. However, Doe et al. (1983) reported pronounced atrophy of the seminiferous tubules in rats exposed to 933 mg 2-ME/m^3 or more (6 h/day, 5 days/week) for 13 weeks. The NOEL was 311 mg/m^3 (Miller et al., 1983b). Studies were also carried out in rabbits, using exposure levels of 93.3, 311, and 933 mg/m^3 (6 h/day, 5 days/week), and most animals exposed to 311 mg/m^3 showed reduced testis size and severe degenerative changes in the tubules. Reduced testis weight was also seen in two out of five animals exposed to 93.3 mg/m^3, and one animal showed histological changes in the germinal epithelium. A NOEL could not be identified, but 93.3 mg/m^3 was near the minimal effective dose in rabbits.

In addition, an increased incidence of sperm abnormalities (principally sperm with banana shaped or amorphorous heads) has been noted in mice exposed to 1555 mg 2-ME/m^3 (7 h per day for 5 days) but not to 78 mg per m^3 (McGregor et al., 1983).

8.5.2 Embryotoxicity and developmental effects

8.5.2.1 2-Methoxyethanol

2-ME has been shown to lead to embryotoxic and developmental effects in laboratory animals following inhalation, oral, or dermal exposure. The effects of 2-ME exposure over the entire organ-forming period of gestation have been studied in rabbits, rats, and mice, the rabbit being the most sensitive species.

The embryotoxicity of 2-ME after gastric intubation was evaluated in mice (31.25, 62.5, 125, 250, 500, or 1000 mg/kg body weight) on days 7-14 of gestation (Nagano et al., 1981). No maternal deaths were observed, but maternal weight gain was reduced in the mice that received doses of 250 mg/kg per day or more. Maternal toxicity was not seen at 123 mg/kg or less. On day 18 of gestation, fetuses were examined and an increase in fetal death rate was observed at doses of 250 mg/kg or more. At doses of 500 and 1000 mg per kg, all fetuses were dead at caesarean section, except for one in the 500-mg/kg group. Approximately 44% (57/130) of the live fetuses in the 250-mg/kg group were found to have gross anomalies, including exencephaly (24), umbilical hernia (3), and abnormal digits (29). One fetus had both exencephaly and abnormal digits. The lone surviving fetus in the 500-mg/kg group had exencephaly and abnormal digits. Minimal skeletal malformations were also observed at the lowest dose of 31.25 mg/kg body weight (a maternally non-toxic dose). Thus, a NOEL could not be ascertained.

Dose-dependent electrocardiographic changes were detected on gestation day 20 in the rat fetuses of mothers exposed orally to 2-ME (0, 25, or 50 mg/kg body weight) on days 7 to 13 of gestation (Toraason et al., 1985). Cardiovascular malformations were observed, including right ductus arteriosus and ventricular septal defects. QRS intervals were significantly prolonged, particularly in the highest dose group, suggesting intra-ventricular conduction delays.

Ornithine decarboxylase (ODC) activity is highest during rapid growth and development in fetuses and is sensitive to maternal exposure to chemicals and drugs. Toraason et al. (1986a,b) evaluated the effect on ODC activity in the fetuses of pregnant rats that received 25 mg 2-ME/kg by gavage during gestation days 7-13 or 13-19. The activity was most affected in fetuses exposed during gestation days 7 to 13. It was highest in 3-day old rats and declined sharply thereafter. No functional or morphological effects were observed in fetuses exposed at maternal dose levels of 25 mg/kg during gestation days 7-13 or in fetuses exposed at that level during days 13-19.

Nelson et al. (1984a) treated male rats by inhalation (78 mg 2-ME/m^3 for 7 h/day, 7 days/week for 6 weeks) and subsequently bred these to untreated females. In addition, groups of 15 pregnant rats were treated with the same dose (7 h/day on gestation days 7-13 or 14-20) and allowed to deliver and rear their young. Neuromotor function activity and simple learning ability were assessed on days 10-90 after birth. Offspring from dams treated between gestation days 7-13 showed significant changes in avoidance conditioning, and changes in neurochemical levels were observed in the brains of 21-day-old offspring from the paternally exposed group as well as from both maternally exposed groups.

8.5.2.2   2-Ethoxyethanol

A dose-finding study in pregnant rats revealed that no offspring survived inhalation exposures of 3312 mg 2-EE per m^3, 7 h/day, during gestation days 7-13 or 14-20 (Nelson et al., 1981). The authors reported 34% neonatal deaths at 736 mg/m^3 under similar exposure conditions. Offspring from dams exposed to 368 mg/m^3 on gestation days 7-13 or 14-20 showed impaired performance in behavioural tests and neurochemical alterations in brain samples.

Using inhalation exposures of 478, 1435, and 2208 mg 2-EE/m^3 on gestation days 7-15 (7 h/day), Nelson et al. (1984b) reported complete resorption of all rat fetuses at 2208 mg/m^3, reduced fetal weight at 1435 mg/m^3, and a

NOEL of 478 mg/m^3. Andrew & Hardin (1984), exposed pregnant rats to 733 and 2823 mg/m^3 for 7 h/day throughout gestation and observed increased fetal resorptions at 733 mg/m^3 as well as skeletal and cardiovascular abnormalities. At 2823 mg/m^3 the resorption frequency reached 100%.

Developmental toxicity has been noted in rats after dermal application of 2-EE (0.25 or 0.5 ml, four times per day) (Hardin et al., 1982) or 2-EEA (0.35 ml, four times per day) (Hardin et al., 1984) on gestation days 7-16. Increased resorption rates and fetal deaths, decreased viable fetus weights, and increased cardiovascular defects and skeletal malformations were seen, even at the lowest dose tested.

The effect of simultaneous administration of ethanol (10% in drinking water) and 2-EE (368 mg/m^3 by inhalation) has been investigated, in view of their related metabolism (via the enzyme alcohol dehydrogenase) (Nelson et al., 1982, Nelson et al., 1984c). Although the results obtained are difficult to interpret, ethanol administration early in gestation tended to reduce the behavioural effects induced by 2-EE, whereas ethanol given late in gestation enhanced these effects.

8.5.3 Teratogenicity

8.5.3.1 2-Methoxyethanol

The teratogenic potential of dermally administered 2-ME was estimated in pregnant rats with the Chernoff-Kavlock screening test (Wickramaratne, 1986). Various concentrations (0, 3, 10, 30, or 100%) of 2-ME in physiological saline were applied to shaved skin and occluded for 6 h of exposure on gestation days 6-17. Animals were permitted to have their litters and rear the pups until 5 days postpartum, when the study was terminated. No adverse effects were noted at the 3% dose level. Small litter sizes and decreased fetal survival were observed at the 10% level. At 30%, lethality was observed in all fetuses, and all pregnant females died when exposed dermally to 100% 2-ME.

The teratogenicity of 2-ME in mice, rats, and rabbits has been evaluated by Hanley et al., (1984). Pregnant rats and rabbits were exposed by inhalation to 0, 9, 31, or 156 mg/m^3 for 6 h/day on gestation days 6-18 (rabbits) or 6-15 (rats), and mice were exposed to 0, 31, or 156 mg per m^3 for 6 h/day on days 6-15 of gestation. No teratogenic effects were found in CF-1 mice and Fischer-344 rats under the conditions of this study, although slight fetotoxicity was noted in both species. In New Zealand white rabbits exposed to 156 mg/m^3 there was a significant increase in resorption rate and incidence of malformations involving all organ systems, as well as a significant decrease in mean fetal body weight when compared to controls. Of the fetuses from dams exposed to 156 mg per m^3, 63% exhibited at least one malformation and 91% of the litters had at least one fetus with a malformation. There were no teratogenic or fetotoxic effects in any of the three species evaluated at 31 mg/m^3.

Developmental phase-specific and dose-related teratogenic anomalies in CD-1 mice resulting from 2-ME exposure have been evaluated (Horton et al., 1985). 2-ME was administered by gavage to pregnant females at doses of 250 mg per kg (during gestation days 7 to 9, 8 to 10, or 9 to 11; during days 7 to 8, 9 to 10, or 10 to 11; or once a day on gestation days 9, 10, 11, 12, or 13) in order to identify the most sensitive developmental phases for the anomalies under study. Resulting malformations were specifically related to the developmental stage at the time of exposure, with exencephaly being observed between days 7 to 10 and paw anomalies (syndactyly, oligodactyly, and stunted digit number 1) during the later stages of development (days 9-12). The dose dependency of digit malformation was studied by administering single doses by gavage (100, 175, 250, 300, 350, 400, or 450 mg 2-ME/kg) on gestation day 11. Dose-related paw malformations were noted in all litters, with forepaws being more susceptible than hindpaws in terms of the number and severity of malformations. At 175 mg/kg digit anomalies were induced without concurrent reductions in fetal weight, while at 250 mg/kg or more digit anomalies occurred concurrently with reduced fetal body weight. In this study, the NOEL for the single exposure (day 11) was 100 mg/kg. Although in this same strain of mice digital malformations were not detected in near-term fetuses given 100 mg 2-ME/kg body weight by gavage on gestation day 11 (Greene et al., 1987), there was a slight increase in the amount of cell death in approximately 50% of the limb buds from embryos collected 24 h after dosing.

In a preliminary study, the teratogenic potential of 2-ME was determined in *Cynomolgus* monkeys using doses of 0.16, 0.32, and 0.47 mmol/kg administered by gavage throughout the period of organogenesis (Scott et al., 1987). Fetal death was dose-related (2/13 at 0.16 mmol per kg; 3/10 at 0.32 mmol/kg; and 8/8 at 0.47 mmol/kg). At the highest dose level, four fetuses were lost through abortion and one of the remaining four, which was re-covered by hysterotomy, demonstrated malformation (ectro-dactyly) of the forelimbs. The MAA content of maternal sera was followed throughout the treatment period. By the 25th day of treatment, MAA levels had more than doubled in all treatment groups, compared to the values determined on day one, indicating that multiple exposure to 2-ME can lead to accumulation of the potentially embryotoxic metab-olite MAA, the possible causative factor in the embryonic deaths and teratogenicity observed (see section 8.8).

8.5.3.2 2-Ethoxyethanol and 2-Ethoxyethanol acetate

Andrew & Hardin (1984) have studied the teratogenic potential of 2-EE in rats and rabbits. Rats (29-38 per group) were exposed by inhalation to 0, 552, or 2388 mg per m^3 5 days per week for 3 weeks immediately prior to mating and then to 0, 743, or 2823 mg/m^3 for 7 h/day from gestation day 1 to 19. Pregnant rabbits received 589 or 2271 mg/m^3 for 7 h/day from gestation day 1 to 18. In the New Zealand white rabbits exposed to 2271 mg/m^3, the rate of early resorptions was 100%. Even at 689 mg/m^3, the number of early resorptions per litter was 6 times that in the control group. There was no evidence of severe intra-uterine growth retardation in surviving fetuses, but a significant increase in the incidence of major malfor-mations (ventral wall defects and fusion of the aorta with the pulmonary artery), minor anomalies, and skeletal vari-ants. Teratogenic effects of 2-EE and also 2-EEA were re-ported in Dutch Belted Rabbits after inhalation exposures of 644 mg 2-EE/m^3 and 2160 mg 2-EEA/m^3 (Doe, 1984a). In this study the author considered the NOEL in rabbits to be 184 mg/m^3 for 2-EE and 135 mg/m^3 for 2-EEA.

In the study by Andrew & Hardin (1984), the highest 2-EE dose (2823 mg/m^3) in rats led to 100% resorption, as in rabbits. The resorption rate per litter in the group gestationally exposed to 743 mg/m^3 was about twice the control value. Fetal body size was significantly decreased, indicating retardation of intrauterine growth. The significant increase in the incidence of cardiovascular defects (transposed and retrotracheal pulmonary artery) and the increased incidence of common skeletal variants and anomalies over control values were indicative of a teratogenic effect of 2-EE in rats. Doe (1984a) reported fetotoxicity without teratogenicity in rats after inhalation exposure to 184 and 920 mg/m^3, but no adverse effects were reported after exposure to 37 mg/m^3.

The teratogenic potential of 2-EE was evaluated in pregnant Sprague-Dawley rats using dermal application (0.25 or 0.50 ml, four times/day during gestation days 7 to 16) (Hardin et al., 1982). No signs of maternal toxicity were noted except for ataxia on the last day of dosing in the high-dose group, as well as a significant decrease in body weight gain in the last half of gestation. All fetuses in the high-dose group suffered intrauterine death. In the low-dose group, there was a significant increase in the number of females with 100% dead implants (p < 0.001), and in the incidence of skeletal variations (p < 0.05). Also, reductions in fetal body weight (p < 0.001) and cardiovascular malformations (p < 0.05) were observed, as were significant decreases in the number of live fetuses per litter (p < 0.001).

Hardin et al. (1984) studied the developmental toxicity of 2-EEA in rats after dermal application of 0.35 ml 2-EEA four times per day on days 7 to 16 of gestation (daily application 1.37 g). 2-EEA was strongly embryotoxic, as reflected by significantly increased frequencies of completely resorbed litters and dead implants per litter. Also, the body weight of live fetuses was reduced relative to water-treated controls. The spectrum and frequency of malformations and variations noted in 2-EEA-treated animals was similar to that described by Hardin et al. (1982) in a previous study.

The developmental toxicity (including teratogenicity) of 2-EEA in rats and rabbits following inhalation exposure has been evaluated by Tyl et al. (1988). Fischer 344 rats (30 animals/group) and New Zealand white rabbits (24 animals/group) were exposed to 2-EEA concentrations of 0, 270, 540, 1080, or 1620 mg/m^3, 6 h/day on gestational days 6-15 (rats) and 6-18 (rabbits). Fetuses were examined for external, visceral, and skeletal malformations and variations on gestational day 21 (rats) and 29 (rabbits). In both rats and rabbits, maternal toxicity and developmental toxicity were observed at exposures of 540 mg/m^3 or more. Teratogenic responses were increased at 1080 and 1620 mg/m^3 with a 100% incidence of total malformations being observed at the highest dose. An exposure of 270 mg per m^3 was considered a NOEL in both species, no evidence of maternal or developmental toxicity being reported at this dose.

8.6   Mutagenicity and Related End-Points

The only published data on 2-EE concerns a point mutation test using *Escherichia coli*, which was reported to be negative (Szybalski, 1958). However, 2-ME has been tested in several *in vitro* and *in vivo* systems for its genotoxic potential. The mutagenicity of 2-ME has been evaluated in the following test systems: Salmonella typhimurium, unscheduled DNA synthesis (UDS) in human embryo fibroblasts, bone marrow metaphase analysis in male and female rats, dominant lethality in male rats, and a sex-linked recessive lethal test in *Drosophila melanogaster*. No evidence of mutagenicity in S. typhimurium was found using five strains, with and without metabolic activation, and dose levels up to 33 mg 2-ME per plate. When 2-ME was tested in the presence of alcohol dehydrogenase no evidence was found that metabolites of 2-ME were mutagenic in S. typhimurium. Similarly, the addition of 2-ME at concentrations up to 10 mg/ml of medium did not lead to changes in UDS in human embryo fibroblasts (McGregor et al., 1983).

The production in CHO cells of sister chromatid exchanges (SCEs) and chromosome aberrations by 2-EE was studied by Galloway et al. (1987). Both assays were carried out with and without activation by an exogenous enzyme system from rat liver chemically induced with the PCB mixture Aroclor 1254. Aberrations were found only in the absence of metabolic activation when using 2-EE concentrations between 4780 and 9510 µg/ml of medium. The lowest effective concentration was 6830 µg/ml. SCEs were found with and without activation, the lowest effective concentration being 3170 µg/ml when the range studied was 951-9510 µg/ml.

Aneuploidy was induced in the diploid yeast strain D61.M (*Saccharomyces cerevisiae*) at 2-MEA levels of 3-5.7% in the medium (Zimmermann et al., 1985). However, there were no chemically related effects in this yeast strain on point mutation or recombination after exposure to 2-MEA. The relevance to mammals of these findings in yeast is not clear.

No statistically significant increase in chromosome aberrations was seen in male or female rats after exposure by inhalation to 2-ME (78 or 1555 mg/m^3), 7 h/day, for 1 or 5 days. Where possible 50 metaphases per rat were scored from groups of 10 animals (McGregor et al., 1983). Basler (1986) dosed Chinese hamsters intraperitoneally (10 animals) with two thirds of the LD$_{50}$ of 2-MEA (approximately 1333 mg/kg body weight in corn oil) and the animals were sacrificed 12, 24, 48, and 72 h after the single dose. No statistically significantly increase in micronucleated erythrocytes was noted.

Two dominant lethal studies in rats have been carried out using 2-ME. McGregor et al. (1983) exposed groups of 10 male CD rats by inhalation to 78 or 1555 mg/m^3, 7 h per day, for 5 days. Control and low-dose groups gave similar results, but the results at 1555 mg/m^3 were difficult to interpret. A high proportion of early deaths was noted, which could be partly explained in terms of the low implantation frequency reported. Therefore, a dominant lethal effect at 1555 mg/m^3 could not be demonstrated conclusively. Rao et al. (1983), using male Sprague-Dawley rats exposed to 93, 311, or 933 mg 2-ME/m^3 by inhalation 6 h/day, 5 days/week for 13 weeks, found no dominant lethal effect at 93 or 311 mg/m^3. An assessment of dominant lethality was impossible at 933 mg/m^3 due to almost complete infertility. No positive control was included.

In a sex-linked recessive lethal test in *Drosophila melanogaster* reported by McGregor et al. (1983), the results were inconclusive. Given the low absolute number of mutants (low sample size), the inconsistency with which various broods were affected, and the lack of a dose-response relationship, a firm conclusion on the mutagenicity of 2-ME in *D. melanogaster* cannot be made.

8.7   Carcinogenicity

No carcinogenicity data are available on these glycol ethers.

8.8   Mechanism of Toxicity - Mode of Action

The metabolic fate of 2-ME, 2-EE, and their acetates has been well studied in both animals (Miller et al., 1983a; Moss et al., 1985) and man (NIOSH, 1986, Groeseneken et al., 1987, Veulemans, 1987a). Due to rapid hydrolysis of the acetates to the monoalkyl glycol ether (see section 6), the putative toxic metabolite are the same for 2-ME or 2-MEA and for 2-EE or 2-EEA.

Both *in vitro* and *in vivo* studies have supported the hypothesis that the toxic effects of 2-ME and 2-EE are elicited by the toxicity of 2-methoxyacetaldehyde and methoxyacetic acid (MAA) from 2-ME and ethoxyacetaldehyde and ethoxyacetic acid (EAA) from 2-EE.

Gray et al. (1985) studied the effects *in vitro* of 2-ME, 2-EE, MAA, and EAA on mixed cultures of Sertoli and germ cells from rat testes. At concentrations up to 50 mmol/litre medium, no morphological damage was noted for 2-ME or 2-EE, whereas administration of MAA or EAA at 2-10 mmol/litre led to degeneration of the pachytene and dividing spermatocytes, the probable target cells of the parent ethers *in vivo* (Chapin et al., 1985b, Creasy et al., 1985; Foster et al., 1986, Oudiz and Zenick, 1986). Foster et al. (1986) reported that 2-methoxyacetaldehyde (2-MALD), a possible metabolite of 2-ME, can produce specific testicular effects *in vitro* and *in vivo* at doses much lower than those required for MAA (0.2 and 0.5 mmol per litre *in vitro*). In more recent studies, Foster et al. (1987) compared the *in vivo* and *in vitro* testicular effects of MAA and EAA in rats. Single oral doses of MAA and EAA (equimolar with 100, 250, or 500 mg 2-ME/kg body weight) were administered and cell morphology was monitored for 14 days. MAA produced damage to spermatocytes undergoing meiotic maturation and division within 24 h of treatment, whereas EAA produced these changes only at the highest dose. Similar results were seen *in vitro* at a dose (5 mmol/litre medium) equivalent to the steady state plasma level of MAA after administration of 500 mg/kg. Evidence that MAA is important in causing 2-ME terato- genicity was reported by Yonemoto et al. (1984). MAA, but not 2-ME, was found to interfere with organogenesis when the two compounds were investigated using rat embryos in culture.

Results from *in vivo* studies in mice (Welsch et al., 1987; Sleet et al., 1988) and rats (Ritter et al., 1985) further substantiate the hypothesis that monoalkyl glycol ethers are metabolized to acetic acid metabolites via alcohol dehydrogenase (ADH) and aldehyde dehydrogenases, and that the ultimate toxin is actually the alkoxy acid metabolite of the glycol ether or a further metabolite. In mice (Sleet et al., 1987), 2-ME and MAA were equipotent in producing teratogenic lesions leading to malformations of the digits of all paws. Similar effects were noted by Brown et al. (1984) and Ritter et al. (1985) in rats. Sub- sequent work showed that the embryotoxic and teratogenic effects of 2-ME in mice could be prevented by the concomi- tant administration of 0.12 or 1.2 mmol/kg of 4-methyl- pyrazole, an inhibitor of ADH, but that 4-methylpyrazole was without effect after the administration of MAA (Sleet et al., 1988).

9. EFFECTS ON MAN

Only limited information on the toxic effects of glycol ethers in humans is available. This information comes largely from case reports in the early literature dealing with accidental poisoning and/or workplace exposure. Such reports provide only minimal information relating specific effects to exposure levels. Only a few epidemiological studies have been reported.

9.1 General Population Exposure

The widespread use of consumer products such as paints, stains, inks, lacquers, surface coatings, and home/industrial cleaners that contain one or more glycol ethers means that broad segments of the general population could be exposed. However, no reports quantifying such exposures have been found nor any that describe skin irritation or sensitization from exposures to glycol ethers in humans, despite widespread exposure.

9.1.1 Poisoning reports

A 44-year-old man consumed 400 ml of 2-ME mixed with brandy and died without regaining consciousness 5 h after he was admitted to hospital in a comatose state (Young & Woolner, 1946). Postmortem findings included acute haemorrhagic gastritis, fatty degeneration of the liver, and black coloured kidneys with marked degenerative changes in the renal tubules.

Two non-fatal cases of poisoning by 2-ME in men aged 41 and 23 were reported by Nitter-Hauge (1970). Both patients consumed 100 ml 2-ME. In addition to nervous system disorders (agitation, confusion), the predominant clinical features were nausea, cyanosis, hyperventilation, slight tachycardia, and metabolic acidosis. In one patient there were suggestions of moderate kidney failure. No evidence of liver damage was found and both patients recovered within 4 weeks.

Ingestion of approximately 40 ml 2-EE by a 44-year-old women led to vertigo, unconsciousness, effects on the central nervous system, and metabolic acidosis (Fucik, 1969). She recovered within 44 days from all symptoms, including kidney insufficiency and signs of liver damage, although neurasthenia was still evident at that time.

9.2 Occupational Exposure

9.2.1 Repeated exposure

Reports on the effects of glycol ethers on humans following repeated exposure are available from occupational studies. Early reports provided evidence that the repeated exposure of humans to solvents containing 2-ME resulted in such effects as anaemia, leucopenia, lethargy, general weakness, dizziness, ataxia, and unequal or exaggerated reflexes. A diagnosis of toxic encephalopathy was made by Donley (1936) and Parson & Parsons (1938), but no reliable estimation of exposure to 2-ME was given. Greenburg et al. (1938) reported levels of 2-ME between 78 and 236 mg per m^3 in one manufacturing plant where 19 male subjects (ages 16-26) were examined. The median duration of exposure was 5 weeks and the maximum was 2 years. Signs of nervous system dysfunction (fatigue, hand tremor, and lethargy) were found, but no clear relationship between the incidence of symptoms and the duration of exposure could be ascertained in this small population. No control group was included in this study.

The development of macrocytic anaemia has been described in a case report of a worker exposed to 2-ME and other solvents during microfilm manufacturing. Exposure to 2-ME averaged 109 mg/m^3 (35 ppm) (56-180 mg/m^3, 18-58 ppm), to methyl ethyl ketone 1-5 ppm, and to propylene glycol monomethyl ether 4-13 ppm for a duration of 20 months. Follow-up analyses conducted 1 month after terminating exposure indicated a return to normal limits for all haematological parameters studied (Cohen, 1984).

The haematological effects of glycol ethers on humans have also been documented in workplace surveys. Obvious symptoms are not always manifested in peripheral blood. The evaluation in a printing plant of seven workers with dermal and respiratory exposure to dipropylene glycol monomethyl ether, ethylene glycol monoethyl ether, and a range of aliphatic, aromatic, and halogenated hydrocarbons used for offset and multicolour printing revealed no alteration in the peripheral blood (Cullen et al., 1983). Although there was evidence of bone marrow injury in three of the seven workers, no direct relationship could be drawn to glycol ether exposure. The exposure to other solvents by this relatively small group of workers makes more definitive conclusions impossible. Bone marrow toxicity had earlier been reported in two case studies of workers exposed dermally to 2-ME (Ohi & Wegmann, 1978).

Denkhaus et al. (1986) investigated the cellular immune response of nine workers aged 25-58 years of age, heavily exposed to mixtures of organic solvents (including 2-ME and 2-EE) for 8-35 (mean 18.9) years, by the analysis of subpopulations of peripheral blood lymphocytes. A control group of matched healthy controls was included. The mean exposures to 2-ME and 2-EE were 6.1 mg/m^3 (peak: 150 mg/m^3) and 4.8 mg/m^3 (peak: 53 mg/m^3), respectively. Based on samples taken during working shifts, mean blood levels were 40.1 μg 2-ME/100 ml (peak: 965 μg/100 ml) and 2.0 μg 2-EE/100 ml (peak: 92.7 μg/100 ml). At these levels (and in the presence of other solvents such as 1-butanol, isobutanol, 2-butoxybutanol, toluene, m-xylene, 2-butanone, and 2-hexanone), the exposed workers had decreased levels of helper T-cells, and increased levels of natural killer cells and human B-lymphocytes. However, the levels of suppressor cells were normal. The authors noted that similar changes in lymphocyte subpopulations are found in states of general immunodeficiency and in immunogenetic forms of aplastic anaemia.

9.2.2 Epidemiological studies

In a cross-sectional study, male employees in a plant manufacturing 2-ME in the USA were examined for haematological effects and possible sterility (Cook et al., 1982). Personal air sampling indicated levels of exposure of 1.3 mg/m^3 or less in one working location and 19-26 mg per m^3 in another. Forty workers, engaged in production and distribution of 2-ME (75% of the possible total population) and 25 controls (57% of total eligible population) were examined for haematological effects, and six exposed and nine control workers participated in an examination of testis size, semen abnormalities, and levels of serum follicle-stimulating hormone (FSH). No increase in the incidence of leucopenia or anaemia was noted, but decreases in white cell count and testicular size were noted in the most highly exposed workers. These results were not statistically significant but correlate with known effects in experimental animals.

A cross-sectional evaluation of semen quality (sperm concentration, pH, volume, viability, motility, velocity, and morphology) was carried out in 37 workers exposed to 2-EE used as a resin solvent in a metal casting plant (NIOSH, 1986). The study population represented 50% of the exposed workforce. A control group of 38 workers from other locations in the plant was included. Full-shift breathing zone airborne exposure to 2-EE ranged from non-detectable to 88 mg/m^3. Dermal exposure was indicated by urinary excretion of EAA at levels from non-detectable to 163 mg/g creatinine. Workers exposed to 2-EE had significantly lower average sperm counts than controls (113 versus 154 million per ejaculate), although both exposed and control groups had lower sperm counts than those found in other occupational groups. The two groups studied did not differ significantly with respect to other semen characteristics or testicular size.

The effect of 2-ME and 2-EE exposure on male reproductive factors and blood has been studied in shipyard painters by Sparer et al. (1988a,b), Welch et al. (1988), and Welch & Cullen (1988). Airborne levels (time-weighted average: TWA) were determined in 102 samples over six workshifts and were 0-80.5 mg 2-EE/m^3 (mean 9.9 and median level 4.4 mg/m^3), and 0-17.7 mg 2-ME/m^3 (mean 2.6 and median 1.4 mg/m^3). Given the methods used by Sparer et al. (1988a,b) the authors concluded these were probably underestimates of exposure, particularly in the mixing room and inside large tanks. Urinary excretion of EAA indicated dermal exposure as well as airborne exposure in some workers. In 73 painters, from a total population of 153, an increased prevalence of oligospermia and azoospermia was noted and there was an increased odds ratio for a lower sperm count per ejaculate in exposed workers as compared to the 40 controls studied (Welch et al., 1988). In addition, when 94 painters from the same population were examined for haematological effects of chemical exposures, 10% were found to be anaemic and 5%

exhibited granulocytopenia (Welch & Cullen, 1988). None of these effects were noted in the 55 control subjects examined. The reproductive effects observed were in agreement with those reported previously by NIOSH (1986).

10. EVALUATION OF HUMAN HEALTH RISKS AND EFFECTS ON THE ENVIRONMENT

10.1 Evaluation of Human Health Risks

10.1.1 Exposure

Many people may be exposed to 2-methoxyethanol (2-ME), 2-ethoxyethanol (2-EE), and their acetates (2-MEA and 2-EEA), at levels comparable to industrial levels, through the use of consumer and trade products. On the other hand, exposure through food, water, or the ambient air is probably negligible. This inference is based only on the physical and chemical properties of these compounds and evidence of rapid environmental degradation.

Significant occupational exposure may occur both through inhalation and skin absorbtion. Limited measurements of air levels in the workplace range from less than 0.1 mg/m^3 to more than 150 mg/m^3. However, the available monitoring is quite limited and large variations may occur both within and among industries. Because of the potential for skin absorption, air monitoring alone may underestimate total exposure. Total uptake may be best estimated from biological monitoring. Occupations where extensive exposure is possible include, for example, painting, printing, and cleaning, but it should be borne in mind that there are many other occupations where these compounds are also used and where exposure is of concern.

10.1.2 Health Effects

The major effects of concern for humans are developmental, testicular, and haematological toxicity. These are demonstrated by extensive and consistent data in animals and some human data. All these effects can be caused by both short-term and longer-term exposures. In experimental animals, very high repeated exposure to 2-ME and 2-EE (over 930 and 1450 mg/m^3, respectively) produces neurobehavioural, hepatic, and renal toxic effects. These are also observed in human poisoning situations.

These four glycol ethers exhibit very similar testicular and developmental toxicities, in all species evaluated, and by all routes of exposure that have been employed (inhalation, dermal, and oral). Mechanistic studies indicate that for both testicular and developmental effects, metabolism to the alkoxyacetic acid derivative is a necessary activation step. Metabolism takes place via the alcohol dehydrogenase system that is common to humans and laboratory animals. The toxic metabolites, methoxyacetic acid (MAA) and ethoxyacetic acid (EAA), have been detected in the urine of humans exposed to these solvents. The consistency of response across laboratory animal species studied, combined with the similarity of metabolism in humans, makes it clear that humans should be presumed to be subject to the testicular and developmental effects of these glycol ethers. Available data on the excretion of alkoxyacetic acids by humans indicate prolonged retention compared with that in laboratory animals, suggesting that humans may be more sensitive than the most sensitive experimental animal species. The rapid skin absorbtion of these compounds is of particular concern. Teratogenicity and other developmental effects have been observed following the application of 2-ME, 2-EE, and 2-EEA to the intact skin of rats.

Testicular damage has been observed in the rat, mouse, and rabbit following exposure to these glycol ethers through both the inhalation and the oral route. Single inhalation exposures of rats to 1944 mg 2-ME/m^3 or more for 4 h and repeated exposure to 933 mg 2-ME/m^3 or more for 13 weeks resulted in histological evidence of testicular damage. The NOEL for acute exposure was 933 mg/m^3 and for repeated exposure was 311 mg/m^3. The mouse appeared somewhat less sensitive, the NOEL for repeated exposure being 933 mg/m^3. However, the rabbit was more sensitive, with marked testicular change being seen after repeated exposure to 311 mg/m^3 and a marginal effect (one in five rabbits affected) being seen at 93 mg/m^3. Similar effects have been seen following oral exposure of rats to 2-ME, with short-term (including single dose) exposure to 100 mg/kg producing testicular damage. The NOEL in a subacute (11 days) study was 50 mg/kg. 2-EE is somewhat less potent with regard to its testicular toxicity than 2-ME;

effects were only seen at dose levels of 500 mg/kg or more, the NOEL being 250 mg/kg.

Evidence from studies in men exposed occupationally to 2-ME and 2-EE is consistent with the animal data and indicates that these glycol ethers can produce testicular toxicity in humans. Epidemiological studies on small groups of workers exposed to 2-EE in a metal casting plant and in shipyard painters exposed to both 2-ME and 2-EE consistently revealed an increased incidence of reduced sperm counts. Data on exposure levels were limited, but there was evidence, in each case, of dermal exposure as well as exposure via inhalation.

Developmental toxicity has been observed in the rat, mouse, rabbit, and monkey following exposure to these glycol ethers using dermal, oral, and inhalation routes. Twelve daily applications of undiluted 2-ME to the shaved skin of pregnant rats (with 6-h occlusion) was lethal, while ten open applications of 2-EE (1.0 ml/day) or 2-EEA (1.4 ml/day) were teratogenic but not maternally toxic. Twelve occluded applications of 10% 2-ME in saline proved developmentally toxic, the NOEL in this study being 3% 2-ME. No-observed-effect levels have not been demonstrated following repeated oral dosing of pregnant animals with 2-ME. The lowest-observed-effect level (LOEL) for oral administration of 2-ME was 31.25 mg/kg per day for mice, 25 mg/kg per day for rats, and 0.16 mmol/kg per day for monkeys. Single-dose studies have been reported only for 2-ME in mice, the results being that on gestation day 11 (the most sensitive day) the NOEL was 100 mg/kg and the LOEL was 175 mg/kg. Both 2-EE and 2-EEA have been evaluated by inhalation exposure in rats and rabbits. Rats were exposed to 2-EE in two studies, resulting in teratogenic effects (743 mg/m^3 for 7 h/day on gestation days 1-19) or fetotoxic effects (184 and 920 mg/m^3 for 6 h/day on gestation days 6-15). In the latter study, the NOEL was 37 mg/m^3. Rabbits exposed to 2-EE also exhibited teratogenic effects (589 mg/m^3 for 7 h/day on gestation days 1-18) or fetotoxic effects (644 mg/m^3 for 6 h/day on gestation days 6-18). In the latter study, the NOEL was 184 mg/m^3. When rabbits were exposed to 2-EEA for 6 h/day on gestation days 6-18, teratogenic effects were seen at 2160 mg/m^3 in one study and 1620 mg/m^3 in another. Fetotoxicity appeared in both studies at 540 mg per m^3 and the lowest exposure level in each study (135 and 270 mg/m^3, respectively) was the NOEL. Rats exposed to 2-EEA by inhalation for 6 h/day on gestation days 6-15 showed the same pattern of response: teratogenic effects at 1620 mg/m^3, fetotoxicity at 1080 mg/m^3, and no effect at 270 mg/m^3.

Thus developmental toxicity has been observed in all species (mice, rats, and rabbits) exposed to 2-ME at 156 mg/m^3 or more. The NOEL for all three species was 31 mg per m^3. Behavioural and neurochemical alterations in rats followed *in utero* exposure at 78 mg/m^3, with no NOEL being identified.

2-EE and 2-EEA were slightly less potent. Developmental effects in rats and rabbits followed all 2-EE exposures at 368 mg/m^3 or more. Slight developmental effects were seen in rats exposed at 184 mg 2-EE/m^3, but 37 mg/m^3 was a clear NOEL. For 2-EEA, the NOEL was 170 mg per m^3 for both rats and rabbits.

Haematological effects from single acute dose exposures have been observed in animals and in human poisonings. Repeated inhalation exposure of the most sensitive species, the rabbit, to 2-ME for 13 weeks, 5 times per week, yielded a NOEL of 93 mg/m^3. Repeat doses of 2-ME also cause haematological toxicity in mice, rabbits, dogs, hamsters, and guinea-pigs. 2-EE is less potent in causing haematological effects than 2-ME. The NOEL for haematological effects in rats and rabbits exposed to 2-EE for 13 weeks, 5 times per week for 6 h/day, is 368 mg/m^3. Dogs and mice also show haematological effects from repeated 2-EE exposure at higher levels. Exposure to the acetate esters of 2-EE and 2-ME would be expected to cause similar effects at similar exposure levels, but there are too few data on exposure and haematological effects of these compounds to determine under what conditions single human exposures will lead to haematological effects.

Industrial exposure levels have been reported at or near the NOEL for haematological effects in animals after repeated doses of both 2-ME and 2-EE. This fact, together with the probable greater sensitivity of humans and the expected accumulation of metabolites in human blood, indicates that haematological effects may well occur from industrial and consumer exposure. This has been confirmed by the haematological effects reported in some of the limited number of studies of industrial workers with repeated 2-EE and/or 2-ME exposure.

10.2   Evaluation of Effects on the Environment

Environmental exposure to these glycol ethers can arise as a consequence of their direct release into the atmosphere from their use as evaporative solvents. Discharges to the land and water from accidental release may also result in environmental exposure. Accumulation in soil and surface water could only occur in the absence of degradation. However, these glycol ethers are rapidly degraded by chemical and biological processes and accumulation is not expected. 2-MEA and 2-EEA are also expected to hydrolyse readily and subsequently biodegrade under aerobic conditions. However, contamination of anaerobic soils and aquifers remains a potential problem, but this condition is expected to be transitory resulting in negligible risk.

Both 2-ME and 2-EE demonstrate low toxicity to microoganisms and aquatic species. The glycol ether acetates, however, are far more acutely toxic. No data exists to ascertain the potential for adverse effects from long-term exposure to environmental species.

11. RECOMMENDATIONS

11.1   Health Protection

1.   Alternative less toxic solvents should be identified to replace 2-methoxyethanol, 2-ethoxyethanol, and their esters, particularly in consumer products. Assessment of the effects of other ethylene glycol ethers is also of particular importance, because some may cause effects similar to the four glycol ethers evaluated here.

2.   In view of the known toxic effects of these glycol ethers, authorities should seriously consider appropriate strategies to alert users of these chemicals to their hazards, particularly those arising from dermal exposures.

3.   In view of recent toxicological data and the potential for considerable dermal absorption of these glycol ethers, national occupational exposure limits should be reconsidered to insure that the total daily dose to workers by all routes of administration does not pose an undue risk to health.

4.   Single dose effects occur in animals at fairly high exposure levels. Prudent use of these compounds (attention to personal hygiene, suitable protective devices, and adequate ventilation) is recommended to reduce the health risks. The data indicate that more extensive protection may be required to prevent developmental effects, as well as effects on blood and testis, from repeated exposure.

11.2   Further Research

1.   In view of the implication of methoxyacetic acid (MAA) and ethoxyacetic acid (EAA) (the principal identified metabolites of 2-ME, 2-EE, and of their esters) in the toxicity to the male reproductive system, their mechanism of action should be investigated. If it transpires that MAA and EAA are not the primary agents concerned, these should be identified and their mechanism of action elucidated.

2. These four glycol ethers are known to have both haematological effects and male reproductive effects (sperm count reduction). The available data, although limited, appear to suggest that the two effects become evident at similar dose levels. The mechanism of action should be investigated for both organ systems, and haematological effects and sperm counts should be examined in parallel to determine if haematological changes offer warning signs for other effects of these compounds.

3. Air monitoring alone is not sufficient to assure low exposure. Biological monitoring can aid in detecting failures in protective measures. At present the relationship between biological indicators of exposure, total body uptake, and observed health effects have not been sufficiently established. Further work is necessary to provide the basis for using biological monitoring in determining safe exposures.

4. Epidemiological studies and/or targeted health surveillance in populations subject to high exposure to these glycol ethers should be designed in order to estimate exposure-effect relationships for the purpose of determining safe exposures, providing that overall exposure can be properly and adequately evaluated by appropriate environmental and biological monitoring.

5. The possibility that these compounds may cause effects on the female gonads should be investigated through multigeneration reproductive studies in animals.

6. Available research indicates that humans may metabolize these glycol ethers to the corresponding alkoxyacetic acids to a greater extent than rats, and that the half-life for urinary excretion of these toxic metabolites is about four times longer in humans than in rats. Furthermore, rats conjugate a large portion of the acid metabolites, whereas humans do not. These differences might contribute to the relatively higher sensitivity of humans to these glycol ethers. Detailed knowledge of the metabolism and excretion kinetics would improve the ability to predict safe exposure levels.

7. The results obtained from short-term (13-week) studies indicate effects on various organ systems. However, there have been no studies of sufficient duration that would

allow the reversibility of such effects to be assessed. Therefore, it is suggested that stop-studies be undertaken in which experimental animals are exposed to these glycol ethers for at least 13 weeks, followed by a suitable recovery period. Important physiological para-meters should then be evaluated in order to determine whether or not these effects are transient.

12. PREVIOUS EVALUATIONS BY
INTERNATIONAL BODIES

Regulatory standards for 2-ME, 2-MEA, and 2-EE, established by national bodies in different countries and the European Economic Community, are summarized in the data profile of the International Register of Potentially Toxic Chemicals (IRPTC, 1987).

REFERENCES

ANDERSON, D., BRINKWORTH, M.H., JENKINSON, P.C., CLODE, S.A., CREASY, D.M., & GANGOLLI, S.D. (1987) Effect of ethylene glycol monomethyl ether on spermatogenesis, dominant lethality, and F_1 abnormalities in the rat and the mouse after treatment of F_0 males. *Teratog. Carcinog. Mutagen.,* 7: 141-158.

ANDREW, F.D. & HARDIN, B.D. (1984) Developmental effects after inhalation exposure of gravid rabbits and rats to ethylene glycol monoethyl ether. *Environ. Health Perspect.,* 57: 13-23.

BAILEY, H.C., LIU, D.H.W., & JAVITZ, H.A. (1985) Time/toxicity relationships in short-term static, dynamic, and plug-flow bioassays. In: Bahner, R.C. & Hansen, D.J., ed. *Aquatic toxicology and hazard assessment: Eighth Symposium,* Philadelphia, American Society for Testing and Materials, pp. 193-212 (ASTM STP 891).

BARBEE, S.V., TERRILL, J.B., DESOUSA, D.J., & CONAWAY, C.C. (1984) Subchronic inhalation toxicology of ethylene glycol monoethyl ether in the rat and rabbit. *Environ. Health Perspect.,* 57: 157-163.

BASLER, A. (1986) Aneuploidy-inducing chemicals in yeast evaluated by the micronucleus test. *Mutat. Res.,* 174: 11-13.

BOTTA, D., CASTELLANI PIRRI, L., & MANTICA, E. (1984) *Ground water pollution by organic solvents and their microbial degradation products,* Luxembourg, Commission of the European Communities, pp. 261-275 (EUR-8518).

BRINGMANN, G. & KUHN, R. (1978) Testing of substances for their toxicity threshold: Model organisms *Microcystis (Diplocystis) Aeruginosa* and *Scenedesmus quadricauda. Mitt. intern. Ver. theor. angew. Limnol.,* 21: 275-284.

BROWN, N.A., HOLT, D., & WEBB, M. (1984) The teratogenicity of methoxyacetic acid in the rat. *Toxicol. Lett.,* 22: 93-100.

CARPENTER, C.P., POZZANI, V.C., WEIL, C.S., NAIR, J.H., KECK, G.A., & SMITH, H.F. (1956) The toxicity of butyl cellosolve solvent. *Arch. ind. Health,* 14: 114-131.

CHAPIN, R.E., DUTTON, S.L., ROSS, M.D., & LAMB, J.C. (1985a) Effects of ethylene glycol monomethyl ether (EGME) on mating performance and epididymal sperm parameters in F344 rats. *Fundam. appl. Toxicol.,* 5: 182-189.

CHAPIN, R.E., DUTTON, S.L., ROSS, M.D., SWAISGOOD, R.R., & LAMB, J.S. (1985b) The recovery of the testis over 8 weeks after short-term dosing with ethylene glycol monomethyl ether: histology, cell specific enzymes, and rete testis fluid protein. *Fundam. appl. Toxicol.,* 5: 515-525.

CHEEVER, K.L., PLOTNICK, H.B., RICHARDS, D.E., & WEIGEL, W.W. (1984) Metabolism and excretion of 2-ethoxyethanol in the adult male rat. *Environ. Health Perspect.*, **57**: 241-248.

COHEN, R. (1984) Reversible subacute ethylene glycol monomethyl ether toxicity associated with microfilm production: a case report. *Am. J. ind. Med.*, **6**: 441-446.

COOK, R.R., BODNER, K.M., KOLESAR, R.C., VAN PEENEN, P.F.D., DICKSON, G.S., & FLANAGAN, K. (1982) A cross-sectional study of ethylene glycol monomethyl ether process employees. *Arch. environ. Health*, **37**: 346-351.

CREASY, D.M. & FOSTER, P.M.D. (1984) The morphological development of glycol ether-induced testicular atrophy in the rat. *Exp. mol. Pathol.*, **40**: 169-176.

CREASY, D.M., FLYNN, J.C., GRAY, T.J.B., & BUTLER, W.H. (1985) A quantitative study of stage-specific spermatocyte damage following administration of ethylene glycol monomethyl ether in the rat. *Exp. mol. Pathol.*, **43**: 321-336.

CREASY, D.M., JONES, H.B., BEECH, L.M., & GRAY, T.J.B. (1986) The effects of two testicular toxins on the ultrastructural morphology of mixed cultures of Sertoli and germ cells: a comparison with *in vivo* effects. *Food chem. Toxicol.*, **24**: 655-656.

CULLEN, M.R., RADO, T., WALDRON, J.A., SPARER, J., & WELCH, L.S. (1983) Bone marrow injury in lithographers exposed to glycol ethers and organic solvents used in multicolor offset and ultraviolet curing printing processes. *Arch. environ. Health*, **38**(6): 347-354.

DAWSON, G.W., JENNINGS, A.L., DROZDOWSKI, D., & RIDER, E. (1977) The acute toxicity of 47 industrial chemicals to fresh and saltwater fishes. *J. hazard. Mater.*, **1**: 303-318.

DE DELBARRE, F., KAHAN, A., DE GERY, A., & KONRAD, K. (1980) Action immunomodulatrice du méthoxy-2 éthanol et de dérivés homologues chez le rat. *C.R. Acad. Sci. Paris*, **291**: 215-218.

DENKHAUS, W., STELDERN, D., BOTZENHARDT, U., & KONIETZKO, H. (1986) Lymphocyte subpopulations in solvent-exposed workers. *Int. Arch. occup. environ. Health*, **57**: 109-115.

DOE, J.E. (1984a) Ethylene glycol monoethyl ether and ethylene glycol monoethyl ether acetate teratology studies. *Environ. Health Perspect.*, **57**: 33-41.

DOE, J.E. (1984b) Further studies on the toxicology of the glycol ethers with emphasis on rapid screening and hazard assessment. *Environ. Health Perspect.*, **57**: 199-206.

DOE, J.E., SAMUELS, D.M., TINSTON, D.J., & WICKRAMARATNE, G.A.D. (1983) Comparative aspects of the reproductive toxicology by inhalation in rats of ethylene glycol monomethyl ether and propylene glycol monomethyl ether. *Toxicol. appl. Pharmacol.*, **69**: 43-47.

DONLEY, D.E. (1936) Toxic encephalopathy and volatile solvents in industry. *J. ind. Hyg. Toxicol.,* **18**: 571-577.

DUGARD, P.H., WALKER, M., MAWDSLEY, S.J., & SCOTT, R.C. (1984) Absorption of some glycol ethers through human skin *in vitro. Env. Health Perspect.,* **57**: 193-197.

ECETOC (1985) *The toxicology of glycol ethers and its relevance to man,* Brussels, European Chemical Industry Ecology and Toxicology Centre (Technical Report No. 17).

FOSTER, P.M.D., CREASY, D.M., FOSTER, J.R., THOMAS, L.V., COOK, M.W., & GANGOLLI, S.D. (1983) Testicular toxicity of ethylene glycol monomethyl and monoethyl ethers in the rat. *Toxicol. appl. Pharmacol.,* **69**: 385-399.

FOSTER, P.M.D., CREASY, D.M., FOSTER, J.R., & GRAY, T.J.B. (1984) Testicular toxicity produced by ethylene glycol monomethyl and monoethyl ethers in the rat. *Environ. Health Perspect.,* **57**: 207.

FOSTER, P.M.D., BLACKBURN, D.M., MOORE, R.B., & LLOYD, S.C. (1986) Testicular toxicity of 2-methoxyacetaldehyde, a possible metabolite of ethylene glycol monomethyl ether, in the rat. *Toxicol. Lett.,* **32**: 73-80.

FOSTER, P.M.D., LLOYD, S.C., & BLACKBURN, D.M. (1987) Comparison of the *in vivo* and *in vitro* testicular effects produced by methoxy-, ethoxy-, and *n*-butoxy acetic acids in the rat. *Toxicology,* **43**: 17-30.

FUCIK, J. (1969) Poisoning by ethylene glycol monoethyl ether. *Prac. Lek.,* **21**: 116-118.

GALLOWAY, S.M., ARMSTRONG, M.J., REUBEN, C., COLMAN, S., BROWN, B., CANNON, C., BLOOM, A.D., NAKAMURA, F., AHMED, M., DUK, S., RIMPO, J., MARGOLIN, B.H., RESNICK, M.A., ANDERSON, B., & ZEIGER, E. (1987) Chromosome aberrations and sister chromatid exchanges in Chinese hamster ovary cells: evaluations of 108 chemicals. *Environ. mol. Mutagen.,* **10**(10): 1-175.

GOLDBERG, M.E., HARN, C., & SMYTH, H.F. (1962) Toxicological implication of altered behaviour induced by an industrial vapour. *Toxicol. appl. Pharmacol.,* **4**: 148-164.

GRANT, D., SULSH, S., JONES, H.B., GANGOLLI, S.D., & BUTLER, W.H. (1985) Acute toxicity and recovery in the hemopoietic system of rats after treatment with ethylene glycol monomethyl and monobutyl ethers. *Toxicol. appl. Pharmacol.,* **77**: 187-200.

GRAY, T.J.B., MOSS, E.J., CREASY, D.M., & GANGOLLI, S.D. (1985) Studies on the toxicity of some glycol ethers and alkoxyacetic acids in primary testicular cell cultures. *Toxicol. appl. Pharmacol.,* **79**: 490-501.

GREENBURG, L., MAYERS, M.R., GOLDWATER, L.J., BURKE, W.J., & MOSCOWITZ, S. (1938) Health hazards in the manufacture of "fused collars". 1. Exposure to ethylene glycol monomethyl ether. *J. ind. Hyg. Toxicol.,* **20**: 134-147.

GREENE, J.A., SLEET, R.B., MORGAN, K.T., & WELSCH, F. (1987) Cytotoxic effects of ethylene glycol monomethyl ether in the forelimb bud of the mouse embryo. *Teratology*, 36: 23-34.

GROESENEKEN, D., VAN VLEM, E., VEULEMANS, H., & MASSCHELEIN, R. (1986a) Gas chromatographic determination of methoxyacetic and ethoxyacetic acid in urine. *Br. J. ind. Med.*, 43: 62-65.

GROESENEKEN, D., VEULEMANS, H., & MASSCHELEIN, R. (1986b) Respiratory uptake and elimination of ethylene glycol monoethyl ether after experimental human exposure. *Br. J. ind. Med.*, 43: 544-549.

GROESENEKEN, D., VEULEMANS, H., & MASSCHELEIN, R. (1986c) Urinary excretion of ethoxyacetic acid after experimental human exposure to ethylene glycol monoethyl ether. *Br. J. ind. Med.*, 43: 615-619.

GROESENEKEN, D., VEULEMANS, H., MASSCHELEIN, R., & VAN VLEM, E. (1987) Ethoxyacetic acid: a metabolite of ethylene glycol monoethyl ether acetate in man. *Br. J. ind. Med.*, 44: 488-493.

GROESENEKEN, D., VEULEMANS, H., MASSCHELEIN, R., & VAN VLEM, E. (1988) Comparative urinary excretion of ethoxyacetic acid in man and rat after single low doses of ethylene glycol monoethyl ether. *Toxicol. Lett.*, 41: 57-68.

GROESENEKEN, D., VEULEMANS, H., MASSCHELEIN, R., & VAN VLEM, E. (1989a) Experimental human exposure to ethylene glycol monomethyl ether. *Int. Arch. occup. environ. Health*, 61: 243-247.

GROESENEKEN, D., VEULEMANS, H., MASSCHELEIN, R., & VAN VLEM, E. (1989b) An improved method for the determination in urine of alkoxyacetic acids. *Int. Arch. occup. environ. Health*, 61: 249-254.

GUEST, D., HAMILTON, M.L., DEISINGER, P.J., & DIVINCENZO, G.D. (1984) Pulmonary and percutaneous absorption of 2-propoxyethyl acetate and 2-ethoxyethyl acetate in beagle dogs. *Environ. Health Perspect.*, 57: 177-183.

HAMLIN, J.W., HUDSON, B., SHEEN, A.D., & SAUNDERS, K.J. (1982) The measurement of glycol ether levels in the workplace. *Polym. Paint Colour J.*, October 13: 61-63.

HANLEY, T.R., Jr, YANO, B.L., NITSCHKE, K.D., & JOHN, J.A. (1984) Comparison of the teratogenic potential of inhaled ethylene glycol monomethyl ether in rats, mice, and rabbits. *Toxicol. appl. Pharmacol.*, 75: 409-422.

HARDIN, B.D. (1983) Reproductive toxicity of the glycol ethers. *Toxicology*, 27: 91-102.

HARDIN, B.D., NIEMEIER, R.W., SMITH, R.J., KUCZUK, M.H., MATHINOS, P.R., & WEAVER, T.F. (1982) Teratogenicity of 2-ethoxyethanol by dermal application. *Drug chem. Toxicol.*, 5(3): 277-294.

6

HARDIN, B.D., GOAD, P.T., & BURG, J.R. (1984) Developmental toxicity of four glycol ethers applied cutaneously to rats. *Environ. Health Perspect.*, 57: 69-74.

HEALTH AND SAFETY EXECUTIVE (1988) *Methods for the determination of hazardous substances: Glycol ethers and glycol acetate vapours in air*, London, UK Health and Safety Executive, pp. 1-7 (MDHS-23).

HERMENS, J., CANTON, H., JANSSEN, P., & DEJONG, R. (1984) Quantitative structure-activity relationships and toxicity of mixtures of chemicals with anaesthetic potency: Acute lethal and sublethal toxicity to *Daphnia magna*. *Aquat. Toxicol.*, 5: 143-154.

HORTON, V.L., SLEET, R.B., JOHN-GREENE, J.A., & WELSCH, F. (1985) Developmental phase-specific and dose-related teratogenic effects of ethylene glycol monomethyl ether in CD-1 mice. *Toxicol. appl. Pharmacol.*, 80: 108-118.

HOUSE, R.V., LAUER, L.D., MURRAY, M.J., WARD, E.C., & DEAN, J.H. (1985) Immunological studies in B6C3F1 mice following exposure to ethylene glycol monomethyl ether and its principal metabolite methoxyacetic acid. *Toxicol. appl. Pharmacol.*, 77: 358-362.

HURTT, M.E. & ZENICK, H. (1986) Decreasing epididymal sperm reserves enhances the detection of ethoxyethanol-induced spermatotoxicity. *Fundam. appl. Toxicol.*, 7: 348-353.

IRPTC (1987) *IRPTC legal file 1986 - Volume 1*, Geneva, International Register of Potentially Toxic Chemicals, United Nations Environment Programme.

JUHNKE, I. & LUDEMANN, D. (1978) The results obtained with the Golden Orfe test during the examination of 200 chemical compounds for acute fish toxicity. *Wasser Abwasser Forsch.*, 11: 161-164.

KAREL, L., LANDING, B.H., & HARVEY, T.S. (1947) The intraperitoneal toxicity of some glycols, glycol ethers, glycol esters and phthalates in mice. *J. Pharmacol. exp. Ther.*, 90: 338-347.

KIRK-OTHMER (1980) *Encyclopedia of chemical technology: Vol. 9 - Ethanol*, 3rd ed., New York, Chichester, Brisbane, Toronto, John Wiley & Sons.

KIRK-OTHMER (1980) *Encyclopedia of chemical technology: Vol. 11 - Glycols (Ethylene and Propylene)*, 3rd ed., New York, Chichester, Brisbane, Toronto, John Wiley & Sons.

LAILLER, J., PLAZONNET, B., LE DOUAREC, J.C., & GONIN, M.J. (1975) Evaluation of ocular irriation in the rabbit: Development of an objective method of studying eye irritation. *Proc. Eur. Soc. Toxicol.*, 17: 336-350.

LAMB, J.C., DUSHYANT, K.G., RUSSELL, V.S., HAMMEL, L., & SABHARNAL, P.S. (1984) Reproductive toxicity of ethylene glycol monoethyl ether tested by continuous breeding of CD-1 mice. *Environ. Health Perspect.*, 57: 85-90.

LAUG, E.P., CALVERY, H.O., MORRIS, H.J., & WOODARD, G. (1939) The toxicology of some glycols and derivatives. *J. ind. Hyg. Toxicol.*, 21: 173-201.

LEE, K.H. & WONG, H.A. (1979) Toxic effects of some alcohol and ethylene glycol derivatives on Cladosporium resinae. *Appl. environ. Microbiol.*, 38: 24-28.

MCGREGOR, D.B., WILLINS, M.J., MCDONALD, P., HOLMSTROM, M., MCDONALD, D., & NIEMEIER, R.W. (1983) Genetic effects of 2-methoxyethanol and bis(2-methoxyethyl)ether. *Toxicol. appl. Pharmacol.*, 70: 303-316.

MELLAN, I. (1977) Glycol ethers and esters. In: *Industrial Solvents Handbook*, 2nd ed., Park Ridge, New Jersey, Noyes Data Corporation, pp. 346-399, 513-551.

MILLER, R.R., AYERS, J.A., CALHOUN, L.L., YOUNG, J.T., & MCKENNA, M.J. (1981) Comparative short-term inhalation toxicity of ethylene glycol monomethyl ether and propylene glycol monomethyl ether in rats and mice. *Toxicol. appl. Pharmacol.*, 61: 368-377.

MILLER, R.R., CARREON, R.E., YOUNG, J.T., & MCKENNA, M.J. (1982) Toxicity of methoxyacetate acid in rats. *Fundam. appl. Toxicol.*, 2: 155-160.

MILLER, R.R., HERMANN, E.A., LANGVARDT, P.W., MCKENNA, M.J., & SCHWETZ, B.A. (1983a) Comparative metabolism and disposition of ethylene glycol monomethyl ether and propylene glycol monomethyl ether in male rats. *Toxicol. appl. Pharmacol.*, 67: 229-237.

MILLER, R.R., AYRES, J.A., YOUNG, J.T., & MCKENNA, M.J. (1983b) Ethylene glycol monomethyl ether. I. Subchronic vapor inhalation study with rats and rabbits. *Fundam. appl. Toxicol.*, 3: 49-54.

MOSS, E.J., THOMAS, L.V., COOK, M.W., WALTERS, D.C., FOSTER, P.M.D., CREASY, D.M., & GRAY, T.J.B. (1985) The role of metabolism in 2-methoxy-ethanol-induced testicular toxicity. *Toxicol. appl. Pharmacol.*, 79: 480-489.

NAGANO, K., NAKAYAMA, E., KOGANA, M., DOBAYASKI, H., ADACHI, H., & YAMADA, T. (1979) Testicular atrophy of mice induced by ethylene glycol monoalkyl ethers. *Jpn. J. ind. Health*, 21: 29-35.

NAGANO, K., NAKAYAMA, E., DOBAYASKI, H., YAMADA, T., ADACHI, H., NISHIZAWA, T., OZAWA, H., NAKAICHI, M., OKUKDA, H., MINAMI, K., & YAMAZAKI, K. (1981) Embryotoxic effects of ethylene glycol monomethyl ether in mice. *Toxicology*, 20: 335-343.

NAGANO, K., NAKAYAMA, E., OOBAYASHI, H., NISHIZAWA, T., OKUDA, H., & YAMAZAKI, K. (1984) Experimental studies on toxicity of ethylene glycol alkyl ethers in Japan. *Environ. Health Perspect.*, 57: 75-84.

NAKAAKI, K., FUKABORI, S., & TADA, O. (1980) An experimental study on percutaneous absorption of some organic solvents. *J. Sci. Labour*, 56(12): 1-9.

NEIHOF, R.A. & BAILEY, C.A. (1978) Biocidal properties of anti-icing additives for aircraft fuels. *Appl. environ. Microbiol.*, **35**: 698-703.

NELSON, B.K., BRIGHTWELL, W.S., SETZER, J.V., TAYLOR, B.J., & HORNUNG, R.W. (1981) Ethoxyethanol behavioral teratology in rats. *Neurotoxicology.*, **2**(2): 231-249.

NELSON, B.K., BRIGHTWELL, W.S., & SETZER, J.V. (1982) Prenatal interactions between ethanol and the industrial solvent 2-ethoxyethanol in rats: maternal and behavioral teratogenic effects. *Neurobehav. Toxicol. Teratol.*, **4**: 387-394.

NELSON, B.K., BRIGHTWELL, W.S., BURG, J.R., & MASSARI, V.J. (1984a) Behavioral and neurochemical alterations in the offspring of rats after maternal or paternal inhalation exposure to the industrial solvent 2-methoxyethanol. *Pharmacol. Biochem. Behav.*, **20**: 269-279.

NELSON, B.K., SETZER, J.V., BRIGHTWELL, W.S., MATHINOS, P.R., KUCZUR, M.H., WEAVER, T.E., & GOAD, P.T. (1984b) Comparative inhalation teratogenicity of four glycol ether solvents and amino derivative in rats. *Environ. Health Perspect.*, **57**: 261-271.

NELSON, B.K., BRIGHTWELL, W.S., SETZER, J.V., & O'DONOHUE, T.L. (1984c) Reproductive toxicity of the industrial solvent 2-ethoxyethanol in rats and interactive effects of ethanol. *Environ. Health Perspect.*, **57**: 255-259.

NIOSH (1986) *Health hazard evaluation report: Precision Castparts Corporation, Portland, Oregon,* Cincinnati, Ohio, National Institute for Occupational Safety and Health (Report No. HETA-84-415-1688).

NIOSH (1987a) Alcohols IV. In: *NIOSH manual of analytical methods,* Cincinnati, Ohio, National Institute for Occupational Safety and Health, p. 1403.

NIOSH (1987b) Esters I. In: *NIOSH manual of analytical methods,* Cincinnati, Ohio, National Institute for Occupational Safety and Health, p. 1450.

NITTER-HAUGE, S. (1970) Poisoning with ethylene glycol monomethyl ether: report of two cases. *Acta med. Scand.*, **188**: 277-280.

OHI, G. & WEGMANN, D.H. (1978) Transcutaneous ethylene glycol monomethyl ether poisoning in the work setting. *J. occup. Med.*, **20**: 675-676.

OUDIZ, D. & ZENICK, H. (1986) *In vivo* and *in vitro* evaluations of spermatotoxicity induced by 2-ethoxyethanol treatment. *Toxicol. appl. Pharmacol.*, **84**: 576-583.

PARSONS, C.E. & PARSONS, M.E.M. (1938) Toxic encephalopathy and "granulopenic anaemia" due to volatile solvents in industry: report of two cases. *J. ind. Hyg. Toxicol.*, **20**: 124-135.

PAUSTENBACH, D.J. (1988) Assessment of the developmental risks resulting from occupational exposure to selected glycol ethers within the semiconductor industry. *J. Toxicol. environ. Health*, **23**: 29-75.

PISKO, G.T. & VERBILOV, A.A. (1988) Toxicity of monomethyl, monoethyl and monobutyl ethers of ethylene glycol. *Gig. Tr. prof. Zabol.*, **3**: 48-49.

PRICE, K.S., WAGGY, G.T., & CONWAY, R.A. (1974) Brine shrimp bioassay and seawater BOD of petrochemicals. *J. Water Pollut. Control Fed.*, **46**: 63-77.

RAO, K.S., COBEL-GEARD, S.R., YOUNG, J.T., HANLEY, T.R., Jr, HAYES, W.C., JOHN, J.A., & MILLER, R.R. (1983) Ethylene glycol monomethyl ether II. Reproductive and dominant lethal studies in rats. *Fundam. appl. Toxicol.*, **3**: 80-85.

RITTER, E.J., SCOTT, W.J., RANDALL, J.L., & RITTER, J.M. (1985) Teratogenicity of dimethoxyethyl phthalate and its metabolites methoxyethanol and methoxyacetic acid in the rat. *Teratology*, **32**: 25-31.

ROMER, K.G., BALGE, F., & FREUNDT, K.J. (1985) Ethanol-induced accumulation of ethylene glycol monoalkyl ethers in rats. *Drug chem. Toxicol.*, **8**(4): 255-264.

ROWE, V.K. & WOLF, M.A. (1982) Derivatives of glycols. In: Clayton, G.D. & Clayton, F.E., ed. *Patty's industrial hygiene toxicology*, Vol. 2, pp. 3909-4052.

SAPARMAMEDOV, E. (1974) [Toxicity of some simple ethylene glycol ethers (single experiments).] *Zdravookhr Turkm.*, **18**(9): 26-31 (in Russian) (English translation from US NIOSH.).

SAVOLAINEN, H. (1980) Glial cell toxicity of ethyleneglycol monomethyl ether vapour. *Environ. Res.*, **22**: 423-430.

SCOTT, W.J., FRADKIN, R., NAU, H., & WITTFOHT, W. (1987) Teratologic potential of 2-methoxyethanol (2-ME) in non-human primates. *Teratology*, **35**(2): 66 (abstract).

SLEET, R.B., JOHN-GREENE, J.A., & WELSCH, F. (1986) Localization of radioactivity from 2-methoxy[1,2-^{14}C]ethanol in maternal and conceptus compartments of CD-1 mice. *Toxicol. appl. Pharmacol.*, **84**: 25-35.

SLEET, R.B., GREENE, J.A., & WELSCH, F. (1987) The teratogenicity and disposition of the glycol ether 2-methoxyethanol and their relationship in CD-1 mice. In: Welsch, F., ed. *Approaches to elucidate mechanisms in teratogenesis*, New York, Hemisphere Publishing Co., pp. 33-57.

SLEET, R.B., GREENE, J.A., & WELSCH, F. (1988) The relationship of embryotoxicity to disposition of 2-methoxyethanol in mice. *Toxicol. appl. Pharmacol.*, **93**: 195-207.

SMALLWOOD, A.W., DEBORD, K.E., & LOWRY, L.K. (1984) Analyses of ethylene glycol monoalkyl ethers and their proposed metabolites in blood and urine. *Environ. Health Perspect.*, **57**: 249-253.

SMALLWOOD, A.W., DEBORD, K., BURG, J., MOSELEY, C., & LOWRY, L. (1988) Determination of urinary 2-ethoxyacetic acid as an indicator of occupational exposure to 2-ethoxyethanol. *Appl. ind. Hyg.*, 3(2): 47-50.

SMYTH, H.F., SEATON, J., & FISCHER, L. (1941) The single dose toxicity of some glycols and derivatives. *J. ind. Hyg. Toxicol.*, 23: 259-268.

SPARER, J., WELCH, L.S., MCMANUS, K., & CULLEN, M.R. (1988a) Effects of exposure to glycol ethers in shipyard painters. I. Evaluation of exposure. *Am. J. ind. Med.*, 14: 497-507.

SPARER, J., WELCH, L.S., SCHRADER, S.M., TURNER, T.W., & CULLEN, M.R. (1988b) Effects of exposure to glycol ethers in shipyard painters. II. Male reproduction. *Am. J. ind. Med.*, 14: 509-526.

STENGER, E.G., AEPPLI, L., MULLER, D., PEHEIM, E., & THOMANN, P. (1971) Toxicology of ethylene glycol monoethyl ether. *Arzneim Forsch.*, 21: 880-885.

STOTT, W.T. & MCKENNA, M.J. (1985) Hydrolysis of several glycol ether acetates and acrylate esters by nasal mucosal carboxylesterase *in vitro*. *Fundam. appl. Toxicol.*, 5: 399-404.

SZYBALSKI, W. (1958) Special microbiological systems II. Observations on chemical mutagenesis in microorganisms. *Ann. N.Y. Acad. Sci.*, 76: 475-488.

TANAKA, K., MIKAMI, E., & SUZUKI, T. (1986) Methane fermentation of 2-methoxyethanol by mesophilic digesting sludge. *J. Ferment. Technol.*, 64(4): 305-309.

TORAASON, M., STRINGER, B., STOBER, P., & HARDIN, B.D. (1985) Electrocardiographic study of rat fetuses exposed to ethylene glycol monomethyl ether (EGME). *Teratology*, 32: 33-39.

TORAASON, M., BREITENSTEIN, M.J., & SMITH, R.J. (1986a) Ethylene glycol monomethyl ether (EGME) inhibits rat embryo ornithine decarboxylase (ODC) activity. *Drug chem. Toxicol.*, 9: 191-203.

TORAASON, M., STRINGER, B., & SMITH, R. (1986b) Ornithine decarboxylase activity in the neonatal rat heart following prenatal exposure to ethylene glycol monomethyl ether. *Drug chem. Toxicol.*, 9(1): 1-14.

TYL, R.W., PRITTS, I.M., FRANCE, K.A., FISHER, L.C., & TYLER, T.R. (1988) Developmental toxicity evaluation of inhaled 2-ethoxyethanol acetate in Fischer 344 rats and New Zealand white rabbits. *Fundam. appl. Toxicol.*, 10: 20-39.

US EPA (1987) *Environmental health criteria: 2-methoxyethanol, 2-ethoxyethanol, and their acetates*, Washington, DC, US Environmental Protection Agency, Office of Toxic Substances.

VERSCHUEREN, K. (1977) Ethylene glycol monomethyl ether. In: *Handbook of experimental data on organic chemicals*, New York, Van Nostrand-Reinhold Company, 327 pp.

VEULEMANS, H., GROESENEKEN, D., MASSCHELEIN, R., & VAN VLEM, E. (1987a) Field study of the urinary excretion of ethoxyacetic acid during repeated daily exposure to the ethyl ether of ethylene glycol and the ethyl ether of ethylene glycol acetate. *Scand. J. Work Environ. Health*, 13: 239-242.

VEULEMANS, H., GROESENEKEN, D., MASSCHELEIN, R., & VAN VLEM, E. (1987b) Survey of ethylene glycol ether exposures in Belgian industries and workshops. *Am. Ind. Hyg. Assoc. J.*, 48(8): 671-676.

WEIL, C.S. & SCALA, R.A. (1971) Study of intra- and inter-laboratory variability in the results of rabbit eye and skin irritation tests. *Toxicol. appl. Pharmacol.*, 19: 276-360.

WELCH, L.S. & CULLEN, M.R. (1988) Effects of exposure to glycol ethers in shipyard painters. III. Hematologic effects. *Am. J. ind. Med.*, 14: 527-536.

WELCH, L.S., SCHRADER, S.M., TURNER, T.W., & CULLEN, M.R. (1988) Effects of exposure to ethylene glycol ethers on shipyard painters: II. Male reproduction. *Am. J. ind. Med.*, 14: 509-526.

WELSCH, R., SLEET, R.B., & GREENE, J.A. (1987) Attenuation of 2-methoxy-ethanol and methoxyacetic acid-induced digit malformations in mice by simple physiological compounds: implications for the role of further metabolism of methoxyacetic acid in developmental toxicity. *J. biochem. Toxicol.*, 2: 225-240.

WERNER, H.W., MITCHELL, J.L., MILLER, J.W., & VON OETTINGEN, W.F. (1943) Effects of repeated exposure of dogs to monoalkyl ethylene glycol ether vapors. *J. ind. Hyg. Toxicol.*, 25(9): 409-414.

WICKRAMARATNE, G.A., de S. (1986) The teratogenic potential and dose-response of dermally administered ethylene glycol monomethyl ether (EGME) estimated in rats with the Chernoff-Kavlock assay. *J. appl. Toxicol.*, 6(3): 165-166.

YONEMOTO, J., BROWN, N.A., & WEBB, M. (1984) Effects of dimethoxyethyl phthalate, monomethoxyacetic acid on post implantation rat embryos in culture. *Toxicol. Lett.*, 21: 97-102.

YOUNG, E.G. & WOOLNER, L.B. (1946) A case of fatal poisoning from 2-methoxy-ethanol. *J. ind. Hyg. Toxicol.*, 28: 267-268.

ZIMMERMANN, F.K., MAYER, V.W., SCHEEL, I., & RESNICK, M.A. (1985) Acetone, methyl ethyl ketone, ethyl acetate, acetonitrile and other polar aprotic solvents are strong inducers of aneuploidy in *Saccharomyces cerevisiae*. *Mutat. Res.*, 149: 339-351.

RESUME ET CONCLUSIONS

1. Identité, propriétés physiques et chimiques, méthodes d'analyse

La présente monographie ne traite que des éthers méthyliques et éthyliques de l'éthylène-glycol, c'est-à-dire le méthoxy-2 éthanol (2-ME), l'éthoxy-2 éthanol (2-EE) et leurs esters acétiques respectifs, à savoir l'acétate de méthoxy-2 éthyle (2-MEA) et l'acétate d'éthoxy-2 éthyle (2-EEA). Ces composés se présentent tous les quatre sous la forme de liquides stables incolores et inflammables, dotés d'une légère odeur éthérée; ils sont tous miscibles à l'eau (ou tout au moins dans le cas du 2-EAA très soluble dans celle-ci) et miscibles à un grand nombre de solvants organiques.

Il existe des méthodes d'analyse permettant la mise en évidence de ces éthers du glycol et de leurs métabolites dans divers milieux (air, eau, sang et urine). Ces méthodes font souvent appel à des techniques d'adsorption ou d'extraction afin de concentrer l'échantillon, suivies d'une analyse par chromatographie en phase gazeuse. La chromatographie en phase gazeuse ou la chromatographie liquide à haute performance permettent de doser l'acide méthoxy-2 acétique (MAA) ainsi que l'acide éthoxy-2 acétique (EAA) (qui sont des métabolites du du 2-ME et du 2-EE) dans les urines, généralement après obtention de dérivés convenables, à des concentrations entre 5 et 100 μg/ml.

2. Sources d'exposition humaine et environnementale

Les quatre éthers du glycol étudiés s'obtiennent tous par réaction de l'oxyde d'éthylène sur l'alcool convenable puis, si nécessaire, par estérification à l'aide d'acide éthanoïque.

On ne dispose pas de données concernant la production mondiale de ces éthers du glycol. Toutefois on peut avancer que la production annuelle globale de l'Europe occidentale, des Etats-Unis et du Japon se situe aux environs de 79 x 10^3 tonnes de 2-ME et de 205 x 10^3 tonnes de 2-EE. Ils sont en grande partie utilisés pour la production industrielle de divers revêtements (peintures, teintures, laques, vernis, etc.) et comme solvants pour la préparation d'encres d'impression, de résines et de colorants, ainsi que pour la fabrication de détachants domestiques et industriels. On les utilise également comme additifs de dégivrage dans les liquides hydrauliques et les carburéacteurs.

3. Transport, distribution et transformation dans l'environnement

Du fait de leur solubilité dans l'eau et de leur tension de vapeur relativement basse, ces éthers pourraient, en l'absence de décomposition, s'accumuler dans l'eau. Toutefois, il semble que cette éventualité soit exclue du fait de leur dégradation par des microorganismes présents dans le sol, les boues d'effluents et l'eau.

C'est l'utilisation de ces éthers comme solvants volatils qui, du fait des émissions atmosphériques auxquelles elle donne lieu, entraîne l'exposition environnementale la plus importante. Dans l'environnement général, ils subissent une photolyse rapide et l'on pourrait s'attendre à des concentrations inférieures à $0,0007$ mg/m^3 (2×10^{-4} ppm).

En aérobiose, les éthers du glycol subissent une dégradation microbienne rapide en dioxyde de carbone et en eau, alors qu'en anaérobiose, les principaux produits finals sont le méthane et le dioxyde de carbone.

4. Concentrations dans l'environnement et exposition humaine

L'utilisation d'éthers du glycol peut entraîner des nombreuses émissions dans l'environnement. C'est en particulier l'exposition humaine directe dans l'industrie, dans les petits ateliers et au cours de l'utilisation domestique de produits à base d'éthers du glycol qui est spécialement préoccupante. En ce qui concerne l'exposition professionnelle, les valeurs signalées vont de concentrations $< 0,1$ mg/m^3 à des concentrations > 150 mg/m^3. L'utilisation de certains produits de consommation à base d'éthers du glycol pourrait provoquer une exposition notable des usagers mais on ne dispose pas de données à ce sujet.

Outre l'exposition par la voie atmosphérique, l'homme peut également être exposé par la voie dermique. L'analyse du sang confirme que ces produits sont rapidement absorbés par cette voie, qui contribue probablement davantage à la charge totale de l'organisme que l'exposition par voie aérienne.

5.   Cinétique et métabolisme

Ces quatre éthers sont rapidement absorbés au niveau de la peau, des poumons et des voies digestives. Des études de répartition portant sur le 2-ME chez des souris gravides ont montré que c'est dans le foie maternel, les voies digestives, le placenta, le sac vitellin et de nombreuses structures embryonnaires que se rencontraient les concentrations les plus fortes.

La métabolisation du 2-ME donne naissance à deux métabolites primaires : le MAA et la méthoxy-2 acétyl-glycine. La transformation en dioxyde de carbone correspond à une voie métabolique secondaire de moindre importance. La conversion plasmatique du 2-ME en MAA s'effectue rapidement, avec une demi-vie de 0,6 heure chez le rat; en revanche l'excrétion de la MAA est lente, sa demi-vie étant d'environ 20 heures chez le rat et de 77 heures chez l'homme.

L'administration à des animaux de laboratoire de 2-EE a conduit à la production d'EAA et d'éthoxy-2 acétyl-glycine, l'EAA étant le principal métabolite qui se manifeste dans l'organe supposé être l'organe cible, à savoir les testicules. Chez l'homme, une étude sur le 2-EAA a permis d'observer une voie métabolique analogue, l'acétate étant d'abord hydrolysé en 2-EE puis oxydé en EAA. Cet EAA a été ensuite excrété avec une demi-vie estimative de 21 à 42 heures. L'expérience semble indiquer que la rétention ou l'accumulation des métabolites pourrait être toxicologiquement importante dans la mesure où ces métabolites seraient responsables de la toxicité observée au niveau de l'organe cible.

6. Effets sur les êtres vivants dans leur milieu naturel

Il semble que le 2-ME et le 2-EE présentent une faible toxicité pour les micro-organismes et les animaux aquatiques. En ce qui concerne les micro-organismes, la concentration létale dans le milieu est supérieure à 2 %. On a constaté une inhibition de la croissance des algues vertes par le 2-ME à la concentration de 10^4 mg/litre et de celle des cyanobactéries (algues bleu/vert) à la concentration de 100 mg/litre. La toxicité aiguë du 2-EE est très faible pour les arthropodes (CL_{50} > à 4 g/litre) et les poissons d'eau douce (CL_{50} > à 10 g/litre). Les acétates des éthers du glycol (2-MEA et 2-EAA) sont beaucoup plus toxiques pour les poissons. Ainsi la CL_{50} du 2-EEA pour le vairon *Pimephales promelas* est de 46 mg par litre tandis que celle du 2-MAA est de 45 mg/litre pour le tarpon et pour *Lepomis machrochirus*. Il n'y a pas eu d'études à long terme.

7. Effets sur les animaux d'expérience et les systèmes d'épreuve *in vitro*

7.1 Toxicité générale

La toxicité du 2-ME et du 2-EE chez l'animal d'expérience a été beaucoup plus étudiée que celle du 2-MEA et du 2-EAA.

En ce qui concerne le 2-ME et le 2-EE ainsi que leurs acétates, la dose létale après exposition unique est du même ordre et ces composés présentent une faible toxicité aiguë, que l'exposition ait lieu par voie dermique, orale ou par inhalation. Pour diverses espèces, les valeurs de la DL_{50} vont de 900 à 3400 mg/kg de poids corporel pour le 2-ME, de 1400 à 5500 mg/kg pour le 2-EE, de 1250 à 3900 mg/kg pour le 2-MEA et de 1300 à 5100 mg/kg pour le 2-EAA. Des valeurs de 4603 mg/m^3 (2-ME) et de 6698 mg par m^3 (2-EE) ont été signalées pour la CL_{50} par inhalation chez la souris.

On ne possède que peu de données concernant les effets irritants au niveau des yeux et de la peau ou le pouvoir de sensibilisation de ces éthers du glycol chez l'animal. Il semblerait qu'ils ne soient pas irritants pour la peau, mais qu'ils puissent l'être pour l'oeil. Chez l'homme, malgré de fortes expositions, on n'a jamais signalé d'irritation cutanée ni de sensibilisation à ce niveau.

On a montré qu'en exposant par voie respiratoire des animaux d'expérience pendant des périodes allant jusqu'à 90 jours, à de fortes concentrations (> 9313mg de 2-ME par m^3 et > 1450 mg de 2-EE/m^3) on déterminait des effets nocifs sur les paramètres hématologiques, le système nerveux, les testicules, le thymus, les reins, le foie et les poumons. A des concentrations plus faibles, les effets ne s'observaient qu'au niveau du système hématopoïétique et des testicules. Par exemple, des rats exposés par inhalation à du 2-ME pendant 13 semaines à des doses comprises entre 93 et 930 mg/m^3, présentaient une réduction de l'hématocrite, du nombre de leucocytes, de l'hémoglobine, des plaquettes et des protéines sériques, mais seulement à la dose la plus forte. Chez des lapins exposés de la même manière, on notait une réduction de la taille du thymus et une altération des paramètres hémato-logiques, à la dose de 903 mg/m^3. Le 2-EE a produit des effets analogues, mais moins graves, chez le rat et le lapin lors d'une exposition de 13 semaines à la concen-tration de 1450 mg/m^3. On ne dispose d'aucune donnée résultant d'études à long terme.

7.2   Cancérogénicité et mutagénicité

On a étudié la mutagénicité du 2-ME sur toute une série de systèmes *in vitro* constitués de bactéries ou de cellules mammaliennes. La plupart des études ont fourni des résultats négatifs, toutefois on a tout de même signalé des résultats positifs à de très fortes concen-trations de 2-ME sur des cellules CHO. Il s'agissait d'aberrations chromosomiques (à des concentrations supéri-eures à 6830 μg/ml) et d'échanges entre chromatides soeurs (à des concentrations supérieures à 3170 μg par ml). La recherche d'aberrations chromosomiques et de micronoyaux n'a rien donné *in vivo*. On ne dispose que de données limitées sur le pouvoir mutagène du 2-EE; en outre, il n'existe pas de données sur la cancérogénicité de ces éthers du glycol.

7.3 Organes mâles de la reproduction

On a étudié de manière approfondie l'effet du 2-ME sur l'appareil reproducteur mâle après administration par voie orale ou respiratoire de ces substances à des rongeurs. La présence de modifications dégénératives au niveau de l'épithélium germinal des tubes séminifères à été systématiquement observée. Des effets analogues ont été constatés avec le 2-EE, mais à des doses un peu inférieures.

L'administration par voie orale à des rats de 2-ME pendant 1 à 11 jours a provoqué une réduction du nombre des spermatozoïdes et des modifications de leur mobilité et de leur morphologie, liées à la dose, à partir de 100 mg/kg de poids corporel. L'autopsie a révélé une atteinte histologique marquée des testicules. La dose sans effet observable (NOEL) était de 50 mg/kg. La réduction de la fertilité était encore manifeste huit semaines après une exposition à 200 mg/kg. Des effets analogues ont été observés dans le cas du 2-EE à des doses supérieures ou égales à 500 mg/kg, administrées pendant des périodes allant jusqu'à 11 jours, la dose sans effet observable sur 11 jours étant de 250 mg/kg. Toutefois l'épuisement des réserves de spermatozoïdes, par suite d'accouplements répétés, s'est accompagné à la dose la plus faible étudiée (150 mg/kg), d'une réduction de leur nombre. Après avoir administré par voie orale à des rats et à des souris une dose unique de 250 mg ou davantage de 2-ME/kg de poids corporel, on a observé chez les animaux une stérilité complète cinq semaines après l'administration, une certaine réduction de la fécondité étant observée dès 125 mg/kg.

L'administration du 2-ME par la voie respiratoire a donné lieu à des modifications dégénératives analogues au niveau des testicules. Les effets en question ont été observés après exposition unique de 4 heures à des doses supérieures ou égales à 1944 mg/m^3, aucun effet n'étant observé à 933 mg/m^3. Les valeurs de la dose sans effet observable étaient de 311 mg/m^3 chez les rats après exposition de 13 semaines (6 heures par jour, 5 jours par semaine) et de 933 mg/m^3 (6 heures par jour) chez les souris après exposition à neuf reprises sur une durée totale de 11 jours. L'exposition de lapins à du 2-ME pendant 13 semaines (6 heures par jour, 5 jours par semaine) a entraîné des effets marqués au niveau des testicules à la dose de 311 mg/m^3 ou davantage; à la dose de 93 mg/m^3, on a observé des effets limites; il n'a pas été possible de déterminer la dose sans effet observable.

7.4   Toxicité foetale

On a observé des effets toxiques sur le développement de plusieurs espèces d'animaux de laboratoire après exposition par toutes les voies possibles, c'est-à-dire orale, respiratoire et dermique. Le 2-ME a produit des effets tératogènes chez la souris, le rat, le lapin et le singe. Le 2-EE et le 2-EEA se sont révélés tératogènes chez le rat et le lapin. Bien que le 2-MEA n'ait pas encore été étudié de ce point de vue, son profil métabolique (voir section 6) incite à penser qu'il a vraisembleblement une toxicité analogue à celle du 2-ME.

C'est dans le cas du 2-ME que l'on possède l'ensemble le plus complet de données dose-réponse (doses de 31,25 à 1000 mg/kg/j). Lors de cette étude portant sur des souris auxquelles le 2-ME avait été administré par gavage (administration les jours 7 et 14 de la gestation), on a obtenu une dose sans effet observable de 125 mg/kg par jour en ce qui concerne la toxicité maternelle. Toutefois des malformations ont été observées à partir de doses quotidiennes de 62,5 mg/kg et des modifications au niveau du squelette à partir de 31,25 mg/kg par jour. La dose sans effet observable relative à la toxicité foetale n'a pas été indiquée. Lors d'études portant sur des doses uniques, des souris ont reçu par gavage du 2-ME au onzième jour de la gestation; la dose de 100 mg/kg n'était pas foetotoxique tandis que celle de 175 mg/kg a produit des anomalies digitales, mais sans autres signes de toxicité maternelle ou foetale. Des anomalis cardio-vasculaires et électrocardiographiques ont été observés chez les rats nouveau-nés après administration les 7ème et 13ème jours de la gestation d'une dose quotidienne de 25 mg/kg. Etant donné qu'il s'agissait de la dose la plus faible expérimentée, l'étude n'a pas permis d'établir une dose sans effet observable sur le foetus (on n'a pas observé de toxicité maternelle à cette dose). De même, aucune dose de ce type n'a pu être déterminée après administration par gavage à des guenons de 2-ME aux doses quotidiennes respectives de 0,16, 0,32, ou 0,47 mmol/kg, du 20ème au 45ème jour de la gestation.

Après exposition par voie respiratoire à du 2-ME à la dose de 156 mg/m³, on a observé une toxicité foetale chez des rats et des souris et des malformations chez des lapins. Pour l'ensemble de ces trois espèces, la dose sans effet observable sur le développement foetal était de 31 mg/m³. Toutefois des anomalies comportementales et neurochimiques ont été observées dans la descendance de rattes exposées du 7ème au 13ème jour ou du 14ème au 20ème jour de leur gestation à une dose de 78 mg de 2-ME par m³.

Après avoir exposé des rats à des doses de 743 mg par m³ de 2-EE et des lapins à des doses 589 mg/m³ de la même substance, on a constaté que ce produit était tératogène (avec en outre une certaine toxicité maternelle). Dans une autre étude, on a constaté une toxicité foetale, mais sans malformations, chez des rats exposés à des doses de 184 ou 920 mg de 2-EE par m³ et chez des lapins exposés à la dose de 644 mg/m³ de la même substance. Pour ce qui est des effets sur le développement foetal, la valeur de la dose sans effet observable était de 37 mg par m³ pour le rat et de 184 mg/m³ pour le lapin. On a observé des anomalies comportementales et neurochimiques dans la descendance de rattes exposées du 7ème au 13ème jour et du 14ème au 20ème jour de leur gestation à la dose de 360 mg de 2-EE par m³.

Des rattes soumises à une application dermique de 0,25 ml de 2-EE non dilué quatre fois par jour du 7ème et 16ème jour de la gestation, ont eu une descendance où l'on notait une foetotoxicité marquée et une forte incidence de malformations malgré l'absence de toxicité maternelle. Des effets analogues ont été observés à la suite d'un traitement indentique par le 2-EEA selon le même protocole au moyen d'une dose équimolaire (0,35 ml, quatre fois par jour).

En exposant par la voie respiratoire des lapines à du 2-EEA du 6ème au 18ème jour de la gestation, on a obtenu au cours de deux études différentes, des réponses tératogènes aux doses de 2176 mg/m³ et 544 mg/m³, la valeur de la dose sans effet observable sur le développement foetal étant respectivement de 135 mg/m³ et 270 mg par m³. L'exposition de rattes du 6ème au 15ème jour de leur gestation à du 2-EEA a entraîné dans leur descendance une toxicité foetale à la dose de 540 mg/m³ et des malformations à la dose de 1080 mg/m³. La dose sans effet observable sur le développement foetal était de 170 mg par m³.

8.   Effets sur l'homme

On ne dispose que de renseignements limités sur les effets toxiques chez l'homme de ces quatre éthers du glycol. Les résultats fournis par quelques études de cas ou études épidémiologiques sur les lieux de travail sont dans la ligne des effets observés chez les animaux de laboratoire. On n'a pas eu connaissance de rapports qui chiffrent l'exposition de la population en général ni les effets sur la santé.

Lors de deux cas non mortels d'empoisonnement par ingestion d'un volume de 100 ml de 2-ME, on a noté les principaux symptômes suivants : nausée, vertiges, cyanose, tachycardie, hyperventilation et acidose métabolique avec quelques signes d'insuffisance rénale. Des sympômes analogues mais moins graves ont été observés chez une personne qui avait ingéré 40 ml de 2-EE. Lors d'un empoisonnement mortel par ingestion de 400 ml de 2-ME, l'autopsie a révélé une gastrite hémorragique aiguë, une dégénérescence graisseuse du foie et une altération dégénérative des tubules rénaux.

L'exposition réitérée de travailleurs à du 2-ME et à du 2-EE, en plus d'autres solvants, a entraîné chez eux de l'anémie, un leucopénie, une faiblesse générale et une ataxie. Dans nombre de ces études, il n'a pas été possible de trouver une estimation fiable de l'exposition des sujets. On a rapporté des effets hématologiques dus aux éthers du glycol chez l'homme et on a notamment décrit l'apparition d'une anémie macrocytaire chez un travailleur exposé à du 2-ME (dose moyenne 105 ml/m³), ainsi qu'à d'autres solvants.

Il a été fait état d'une toxicité médullaire chez des ouvriers dont l'épiderme était exposé à du 2-ME, et des effets immunologiques ont été également notés à la suite d'une exposition prolongée (8 à 35 années) au 2-ME et au

2-EE (doses moyennes d'exposition 6,1 mg/m^3 et 4,8 mg par m^3 respectivement).

Des études épidémiologiques effectuées sur des ouvriers exposés à du 2-ME et à du 2-EE ont révélé des anomalies au niveau de la fonction de reproduction, avec une fréquenc accrue des cas d'oligospermie. L'exposition à du 2-EE (37 ouvriers) à des concentrations pouvant atteindre 88,5 mg/m^3 a entraîné une modification du spermogramme. Parmi 73 ouvriers exposés à du 2-ME (jusqu'à 17,7 mg/m^3) et à du 2-EE (jusqu'à 80,5 mg/m^3), on a constaté une fréquence accrue de cas d'oligospermie et observé certains effets hématologiques, pour des doses d'exposition (TWA) de 2,6 mg/m^3 dans le cas du 2-ME et de 9,9 mg/m^3 dans celui du 2-EE.

Les effets indésirables constatés chez l'homme par suite d'une exposition professionnelle correspondent à ceux qui ont été observés chez les animaux de laboratoire. Cependant, l'évaluation de l'exposition présentant un certain nombre d'insuffisances et du fait qu'il s'agissait d'expositions simultanées à plusieurs substances, il n'a pas été possible d'en déduire une relation dose-réponse.

9. Conclusions

De nombreuses personnes peuvent être exposées à ces quatre éthers du glycol à des concentrations comparables à celles que l'on rencontre dans l'industrie, par suite de l'utilisation de certains produits de consommation ou de produits commerciaux. Une exposition professionnelle non négligeable peut se produire par inhalation ou par résorption cutanée. Des mesures faites en petit nombre dans l'air des lieux de travail indiquent des teneurs allant < 0,1 mg/m^3 à > 150 mg/m^3.

Le 2-ME et le 2-EE sont tous deux d'une faible toxicité pour les micro-organismes et les espèces aquatiques. Il n'existe aucune donnée qui permettrait d'évaluer le risque d'effets indésirables sur les êtres vivants dans leur milieu naturel par suite d'une exposition de longue durée.

Chez le rat, la dose de 2-ME sans effets aigus observables au niveau testiculaire, est de 933 mg/m^3; en cas d'exposition répétée, la dose sans effet observable est de

311 mg/m^3. En exposant de manière répétée l'espèce la plus sensible, à savoir le lapin, on a observé un effet net dès 311 mg/m^3; cet effet était limite à la dose de 93 mg/m^3 (un animal sur cinq). Les données fournies par des études effectuées sur des sujets humains exposés de par leur profession à du 2-ME et à du 2-EE montrent que ces éthers du glycol exercent une certaine toxicité testiculaire.

Chez toutes les espèces étudiées (souris, rats et lapins) on a observé après exposition au 2-ME à des doses égales ou supérieures à 156 mg/m^3, une toxicité vis-à-vis du développement foetal. Des anomalies comportementales et neurochimiques ont été observées chez le rat après exposition *in utero* à 78 mg/m^3 de cette substance sans qu'on puisse déterminer de dose sans effet observable. Le 2-EE et le 2-EEA se sont révélés légèrement moins actifs. Des effets ont été également observés sur le développement de foetus de rats et de lapins après exposition à du 2-EE à des doses égales ou supérieures 368 mg/m^3. Ces effets étaient légers chez les rats exposés à 184 mg de 2-EE par m^3 mais on a pu néanmoins fixer nettement la dose sans effet observable chez le rat et le lapin à la valeur de 38 mg/m^3.

Ces éthers du glycol produisent des effets hématologiques chez la souris, le rat, le lapin, le chien, le hamster et le cobaye. Ces résultats sont en accord avec les anomalies hématologiques observées lors des quelques études consacrées à des travailleurs de l'industrie qui avaient subi des expositions répétées à du 2-EE et/ou du 2-ME. Lors d'études sur l'animal comportant une exposition répétée à ces deux substances, on a fixé à 93 mg par m^3 la dose de 2-ME sans effet observable chez le lapin et à 368 mg/m^3 la dose de 2-EE sans effet observable chez le rat et le lapin. On n'a pas pu obtenir de données qui permettent une évaluation quatitative des effets hématologiques aigus consécutifs à une exposition.

EVALUATION DES RISQUES POUR LA SANTE HUMAINE ET DES EFFETS SUR L'ENVIRONNEMENT

1. Evaluation des risques pour la santé humaine

1.1 Exposition

Nombreuses sont les personnes qui peuvent être exposées au méthoxy-2 éthanol (2-ME), à l'éthoxy-2 éthanol (2-EE) et à leurs acétates (2-MEA et 2-EEA) à des concentrations comparables à celles que l'on rencontre dans l'industrie, lors de l'utilisation de produits de consommation et de produits commerciaux. En revanche l'exposition par l'intermédiaire des denrées alimentaires, de l'eau ou de l'air ambiant est probablement négligeable. Cette hypothèse ne repose que sur les propriétés physiques et chimiques de ces composés et sur le fait qu'ils se dégradent rapidement dans l'environnement.

Une exposition professionnelle non négligeable peut se produire par inhalation ou résorption cutanée. Les quelques mesures de concentrations dans l'air des lieux de travail ont donné des valeurs qui vont de moins de 0,1 mg par m^3 à plus de 150 mg/m^3. Toutefois les données de surveillance existantes sont très limitées et il peut y avoir d'importantes variations entre les différentes industries et dans une même industrie. En raison du risque de résorption cutanée, une simple surveillance de l'air des lieux de travail risque de sous estimer l'exposition totale. Pour évaluer la charge totale de l'organisme, la meilleure méthode consiste à faire un contrôle biologique. Une forte exposition peut se produire lors de travaux tels que la peinture, l'impression ou le nettoyage mais il faut se souvenir que ces composés sont utilisés à l'occasion d'un grand nombre d'autres activités au cours desquelles on pourrait craindre une exposition.

1.2 Effets sur la santé

Les principaux effets qu'on peut craindre chez l'homme tiennent à l'action toxique de ces composés sur le développement foetal, les testicules et les paramètres hématologiques. La réalité de ces effets est attestée par des données nombreuses et cohérentes obtenues chez l'animal ainsi que par quelques données concernant l'homme. Tous ces effets peuvent apparaître par suite d'expositions à court ou à long terme. Chez l'animal de laboratoire, une exposition répétée à des très fortes doses de 2-ME et de 2-EE (plus de 930 ou 1450 mg/m^3, respectivement) entraîne des effets toxiques qui se traduisent par des anomalies neuro-comportementales, hépatiques et rénales. On les observe également dans les cas d'intoxication humaine.

Ces quatre éthers du glycol exercent des effets toxiques très voisins tant sur les testicules que sur le développement du foetus, et ce, chez toutes les espèces étudiées et par toutes les voies d'exposition qui ont été utilisées (voie respiratoire, voie percutanée, voie orale). L'étude du mécanisme de ces effets montre que dans les deux cas, une phase d'activation est nécessaire, à savoir la métabolisation en un dérivé de l'acide alkoxy-acétique correspondant. La métabolisation s'effectue en présence du système de l'alcool déshydrogénase qui est commun à l'homme et aux animaux de laboratoire. Des méta-bolites toxiques, l'acide méthoxyacétique (MAA) et l'acide éthoxyacétique (EAA) ont été décelés dans l'urine de sujets exposés à ces solvants. La régularité de cette réponse toxique d'une espèce animale à l'autre, jointe à l'analogie du métabolisme chez l'homme et l'animal, montrent à l'évidence que l'homme pourrait être la cible des mêmes effets toxiques sur les testicules et le développement foetal. Les données dont on dispose au sujet de l'excrétion des acides alkoxyacétiques chez l'homme indiquent que leur durée de rétention est plus longue chez celui-ci que chez l'animal, ce qui incite à penser que l'homme pourrait être plus sensible à ces effets que l'animal de laboratoire le plus sensible. C'est la résorption cutanée rapide de ces composés qui est parti-culièrement préoccupante. On a observé des effets térato-gènes et autres anomalies du developpement à la suite de l'application de 2-ME, de 2-EE et de 2-EAA sur la peau intacte du rat.

Des lésions testiculaires ont été observées chez le rat, la souris et le lapin à la suite d'une exposition à ces éthers du glycol, soit par la voie respiratoire soit par la voie orale. Chez le rat, une seule exposition par voie respiratoire à des doses de 2-ME supérieures ou

égales à 1944 mg/m^3 pendant 4 heures et une exposition
répétée à des doses supérieures ou égales à 933 mg par
m^3 pendant 13 semaines ont déterminé des anomalies histo-
logiques au niveau testiculaire. Dans le cas de l'exposition unique, la dose sans effet observable était de 933
mg/m^3; elle était 311 mg/m^3 dans le cas d'expositions
répétées. La souris a semblé un peu moins sensible, la
dose sans effet observable dans son cas étant, pour des
expositions répétées, de 933 mg/m^3. Toutefois le lapin
l'était davantage, avec des altérations testiculaires
marquées qu'on pouvait observer après des expositions
répétées à 311 mg/m^3 et la présence d'effets limites (un
lapin sur cinq) dès la dose de 93 mg/m^3. Des effets analogues ont été observés à la suite de l'exposition par
voie orale de rats à du 2-ME, une exposition de courte
durée (et notamment à une dose unique) ayant déterminé des
lésions testiculaires à partir de 100 mg/m^3. Dans le
cas d'une étude portant sur les effets subaigus (11 jours)
la dose sans effet observable a été de 50 mg/kg. Le 2-EE
présente une toxicité testiculaire un peu moindre que
celle du 2-ME; ces effets n'apparaissent qu'à des doses
de 500 mg/kg ou davantage et la dose sans effet observable
se situe à 250 mg/kg.

Les données fournies par les études menées sur des
sujets humains exposés de par leur profession à du 2-ME et
à du 2-EE cadrent avec les données obtenues sur l'animal
et montrent que ces éthers du glycol peuvent produire des
effets toxiques au niveau testiculaire chez l'homme. Des
études épidémiologiques portant sur de petits groupes de
travailleurs exposés au 2-EE dans un atelier de fonte de
métaux et chez des peintres d'un chantier naval exposés à
ces deux composés, ont révélé une oligospermie systéma-
tique. Les données relatives aux niveaux d'exposition sont
limitées mais dans chaque cas, il y a lieu de penser qu'il
y a eu exposition par voie cutanée et respiratoire.

On a observé chez le rat, la souris, le lapin et le
singe des effets toxiques sur le développement embryonnaire après exposition à ces éthers du glycol par voie
percutanée, orale ou respiratoire. Du 2-ME non dilué
appliqué à 12 reprises au cours d'une journée sur la peau
rasée de rattes gravides (zone d'application couverte
pendant 6 heures) s'est révélé mortel pour les animaux
alors qu'appliqué à 10 reprises sans pansement, du 2-EE

(1,0 ml/jour) ou du 2-EEA (1,4 ml/jour) ont produit des effets tératogènes mais n'ont pas été toxiques pour les femelles gravides. Au cours d'une autre étude, 12 applications de 2-ME à 10 % dans du soluté physiologique, avec pansement sur le site d'application, ont entraîné des effets toxiques sur le développement embryonnaire, la dose sans effet observable se situant à la concentration de 3 %. Après administration répétée par voie orale de 2-ME à des animaux gravides, on n'a pas observé de dose sans effet toxique. La dose la plus faible produisant un effet observable dans le cas de l'administration par voie orale était de 31,5 mg/kg par jour pour la souris, de 25 mg/kg pour le rat et de 0,16 mmol/kg pour le singe. En ce qui concerne l'administration d'une dose unique, on ne possède des résultats que pour le 2-ME chez la souris, avec une dose sans effet observable pour le 11ème jour de la gestation (le jour le plus sensible) de 100 mg/kg et une valeur de 175 mg/kg pour la dose la plus faible avec effet observable. Le 2-EE et le 2-EEA ont fait l'objet d'études au cours desquelles des rats et des lapins ont été exposés à ces deux composés par la voie respiratoire. L'exposition des rats au 2-EE a fait l'objet de deux études qui ont révélé des effets tératogènes (743 mg/m^3, 7 heures par jour, du premier au 19ème jour de la gestation) ou des effets foetotoxiques (184 et 920 mg/m^3, 6 heures par jour, du 6ème au 15ème jour de la gestation). Dans cette dernière étude, on a trouvé une dose sans effet observable de 37 mg/m^3. Chez des lapins exposés à du 2-EE on a également observé des effets tératogènes (589 mg/m^3, 7 heures par jour du premier au 18ème jour de la gestation) et des effets foetotoxiques (644 mg/m^3, 6 heures par jour, du 6ème au 18ème jour de la gestation). Dans cette dernière étude, la dose sans effet observable était de 184 mg/m^3. Chez des lapines exposées à du 2-EEA 6 heures par jour du 6ème au 18ème jour de la gestation, on a observé des effets tératogènes à la dose de 2160 mg/m^3 dans une étude et à la dose de 1620 mg/m^3 dans une autre. Les deux études ont montré l'apparition d'une foetotoxicité à 540 mg/m^3; la dose sans effet observable correspondant, dans chaque étude, à la dose la plus faible étudiée (respectivement 135 et 270 mg/m^3). Des rats exposés par voie respiratoire à du 2-EEA 6 heures par jour du 6ème au 15ème jour de la gestation ont présenté le même de type de réactions : effets tératogènes à 1620 mg par m³, foetotoxicité à 1080 mg/m³ et aucun effet à 260 mg par m³.

Des effets toxiques sur le développement embryonnaire ont donc été observés chez toutes les espèces (souris, rats et lapins), exposées à des doses supérieures ou égales à 156 mg de 2-ME. Pour ces trois espèces, la dose sans effet observable était de 31 mg/m³. Après exposition *in utero* à 78 mg/m³, on a observé chez la descendance des altérations comportementales et neurochimiques sans qu'il soit possible de déterminer la dose sans effet observable.

Le 2-EE et le 2-EEA se sont révélés légèrement moins actifs. Des effets toxiques sur le développement embryonnaire ont été observés chez des rats et des lapins après exposition à des doses supérieures ou égales à 368 mg par m³ de 2-EE. De légers effets de ce type ont été également observés chez des rats exposés à 184 mg de 2-EE/m³, la dose sans effet observable étant clairement établie à 37 mg/m³. En ce qui concerne le 2-EEA, la dose sans effet observable était de 170 mg/m³ pour les rats et les lapins.

Des effets hématologiques consécutifs à une exposition à une dose unique on été observés chez l'animal ainsi qu'à la suite d'intoxications chez l'homme. L'exposition répétée par voie respiratoire, de lapins, l'espèce la plus sensible, à du 2-ME 5 fois par semaine pendant 13 semaines, a permis de fixer la dose sans effet observable à 93 mg/m³. Administré à répétition, le 2-ME produit également des anomalies hématologiques chez la souris, le lapin, le chien, le hamster et le cobaye. Le 2-EE est moins actif à cet égard que le 2-ME. En ce qui concerne les effets hématologiques chez le rat et le lapin, après exposition à du 2-EE pendant 13 semaines, 5 fois par semaine et 6 heures par jour, on peut fixer la dose sans effet observable à 368 mg/m³. Chez le chien et la souris, on observe également après, exposition répétée à des doses plus élevées, un certain nombre d'effets hématologiques. L'exposition aux acétates de 2-EE et de 2-ME devrait provoquer des effets analogues, toutes choses égales d'ailleurs, mais les données dont on dispose sur l'exposition et les effets hématologiques de ces composés sont trop limitées pour qu'on puisse établir les conditions dans lesquelles une seule exposition conduirait à des effets hématologiques chez l'homme.

On a observé dans l'industrie des niveaux d'exposition voisins de la dose sans effet hématologique observable que l'on a pu déterminer chez l'animal après expositions répétées à du 2-ME et à du 2-EE. On peut en conclure, compte tenu de la sensibilité probablement plus grande de l'homme et de l'accumulation vraisemblable de métabolites dans le sang, que l'exposition résultant de l'utilisation de produits de consommation ou d'activités dans l'industrie pourrait entraîner des effets hématologiques de ce genre. A l'appui de cette hypothèse, on peut citer les effets hématologiques effectivement signalés lors de quelques études effectuées chez des travailleurs de l'industrie ayant subi des expositions répétées au 2-EE et/ou au 2-ME.

2.   Evaluation des effets sur l'environnement

La libération directe dans l'atmosphère ou l'utilisation de ces produits comme solvants volatils peut conduire à une exposition dans le milieu ambiant. Ce peut être également le cas par suite d'une libération accidentelle sur le sol ou dans l'eau. L'accumulation dans le sol et les eaux superficielles ne peut se produire qu'en l'absence de dégradation de ces composés. Or, on sait que ces éthers du glycol se décomposent rapidement sous l'effet de processus chimiques et biologiques; ils ne devraient donc pas s'accumuler. Le 2-MEA et le 2-EAA devraient également s'hydrolyser rapidement et subir ensuite une biodégradation aérobie. Toutefois dans des conditions d'anaérobiose, on pourrait craindre une contamination des sols et des nappes phréatiques encore que le phénomène soit vraisemblablement transitoire et le risque correspondant négligeable.

Le 2-ME et le 2-EE sont peu toxiques pour les micro-organismes et les espèces aquatiques. Leurs acétates, en revanche, présentent une toxicité aiguë beaucoup plus forte. On ne dispose pas de données à partir desquelles on puisse déterminer leur potentiel nocif pour les espèces vivantes en cas d'exposition prolongée.

RECOMMANDATIONS

1. Protection de la santé

1 Il conviendrait de recercher des solvants moins toxiques que le méthoxy-2 éthanol, l'éthoxy-2 éthanol et leurs esters, en particulier pour les remplacer dans les produits de consommation. Il est également important d'évaluer les effets des autres éthers de l'éthylène-glycol car certains d'entre eux pourraient excercer des effets analogues aux quatre éthers qui ont fait l'objet de la présente évaluation.

2. Du fait des effets toxiques reconnus de ces éthers du glycol, les autorités responsables devraient se préoccuper sérieusement de trouver les moyens d'avertir les consommateurs des dangers que présente l'utilisation de ces produits, en particulier en cas d'exposition par voie cutanée.

3. Compte tenu des données toxicologiques récentes et de la possibilité d'une très forte absorption percutanée des ces éthers du glycol, il importe de revoir les limites nationales d'exposition professionnelle pour faire en sorte que la dose quotidienne totale à laquelle sont exposés les travailleurs par n'importe quelle voie, ne menace pas leur santé.

4. Lorsqu'elle est assez importante, une dose unique peut produire des effets sur l'animal. Pour réduire les risques, il est recommandé d'utiliser ces produits avec prudence (veiller à l'hygiène personnelle, utiliser des dispositifs protecteurs appropriés et assurer une ventilation suffisante). Les données montrent que les effets toxiques sur le développement embryonnaires ainsi que sur le sang et les testicules, consécutifs à une exposition répétée, pourraient exiger des mesures de protection plus importantes.

2. Recherches à affectuer

1. Du fait que l'acide méthoxyacétique (MAA) et l'acide éthoxyacétique (EAA), qui sont les principaux métabolites du 2-ME, du 2-EE et de leurs esters, exercent des effets toxiques sur les organes reproducteurs mâles, il faudrait

en étudier le mode d'action. S'ils apparaît que le MAA et EAA ne sont pas les véritables responsables de ces effets, ceux-ci devront être identifiés et leur mode d'action élucidé.

2. Ces quatre éthers du glycol ont des effets sur le sang et sur la fonction de reproduction masculine (oligospermie). Les données disponibles, bien qu'en nombre limité, indiquent que ces deux effets se manifestent à des doses analogues. Il faudrait étudier le mode d'action de ces composés sur ces deux types d'organes et étudier parallèlement le nombre de spermatozoïdes et les effets hématologiques afin de voir si ces derniers sont susceptibles de jouer le rôle de signal d'alarme pour d'autres effets toxiques de ces composés.

3. La surveillance de l'air ne suffit pas à assurer une faible exposition. Un contrôle biologique peut permettre de déceler les insuffisances des mesures de protection. A l'heure actuelle on n'a pas établi avec une certitude suffisante la relation qui existe entre les indicateurs biologiques de l'exposition, la charge totale de l'organisme et les effets physiologiques observés. Des travaux sont encore nécessaires pour pouvoir établir les limites de sécurité en fonction des résultats de la surveillance biologique.

4. Il faudrait envisager des études épidémiologiques ou une surveillance sanitaire spécifique au sein de populations qui sont fortement exposées à ces éthers du glycol afin d'obtenir des relations exposition-effets; on pourrait alors déterminer les limites de sécurité, à condition toutefois que l'exposition globale puisse être correctement et suffisamment évaluée par la surveillance de l'environnement et des contrôles biologiques.

5. Il conviendrait d'étudier l'éventualité d'effets sur l'appareil reproducteur féminin en procédant à des études de reproduction sur plusieurs générations d'animaux de laboratoire.

6. Les résultats disponibles indiquent que l'homme pourrait métaboliser dans une plus grande proportion que le rat ces éthers du glycol en acides alkoxyacétiques correspondants, la demi-vie des ces métabolites toxiques s'étant environ quatre fois plus longue chez l'homme. Par

ailleurs l'organisme du rat est capable de conjuguer une fraction plus importante des métabolites acides que ne le fait celui de l'homme. Ces différences pourraient entraîner une sensibilité relativement plus importante de l'homme aux éthers du glycol. Une connaissance plus précise du métabolisme et de la cinétique d'excrétion de ces composés permettrait de mieux prévoir les limites de sécurité.

7. Les résultats fournis par des études à court terme (13 semaines) montrent que des effets s'exercent sur divers organes. Toutefois, il n'a pas été procédé à des études suffisamment longues pour qu'on puisse déterminer si ces effets sont réversibles ou non. Il est donc recommandé de procéder à des études au cours desquelles des animaux de laboratoire subiront une exposition d'au moins 13 semaines à ces composés, suivie d'une période de récupération. A l'issue de cette période, on devra déterminer les paramètres physiologiques importants afin de voir si les effets sont passagers ou non.

RESUMEN Y CONCLUSIONES

1. Identidad, propiedades físicas y químicas, métodos analíticos

En esta monografía sólo se tienen en cuenta los éteres metílico y etílico del etilenglicol, es decir el 2-metoxietanol (2-ME) y el 2-etoxietanol (2-EE), así como sus ésteres acéticos respectivos, el acetato de 2-metoxietilo (2-MEA) y el acetato de 2-etoxietilo (2-EEA). Estos cuatro compuestos son todos ellos líquidos estables, incoloros e inflamables con un olor levemente etéreo y todos ellos son miscibles con (o, en el caso del 2-EEA, muy solubles en) agua y miscibles con numerosos solventes orgánicos.

Se dispone de métodos analíticos para detectar estos éteres glicólicos o sus metabolitos en diversos medios (aire, agua, sangre y orina). En muchos casos se basan en el empleo de métodos de adsorción o extracción para concentrar la muestra, seguidos de un análisis por cromatografía de gases. Mediante la cromatografía de gases o la cromatografía de líquidos de alto rendimiento, cabe la posibilidad de determinar cuantitativamente el ácido 2-metoxiacético (MAA) y el ácido 2-etoxiacético (EAA) - metabolitos del 2-ME y del 2-EE - en la orina, por lo general tras derivación, a concentraciones de 5-100 μg por ml.

2. Fuentes de exposición humana y ambiental

Los cuatro éteres glicólicos examinados están todos ellos producidos por la reacción del óxido etilénico con el alcohol apropiado, seguida, si procede, de esterificación con ácido etanoico.

No se dispone de datos sobre la producción mundial de estos éteres glicólicos. Sin embargo, la producción anual combinada de Europa occidental, los Estados Unidos de América y el Japón es aproximadamente del 79 x 10^3 toneladas de 2-ME y 205 x 10^3 toneladas de 2-EE. Una proporción considerable se utiliza en la fabricación de pinturas, colorantes y lacas así como en forma de solventes para tinta de imprenta, resinas y tintes, y como productos de limpieza domésticos e industriales. También se utilizan estos compuestos como aditivos anticongelantes en los líquidos hidráulicos y el combustible de los reactores.

3. Transporte, distribución y transformación en el medio ambiente

La hidrosolubilidad de estos éteres glicólicos y su presión de vapor relativamente baja podrían dar lugar a su acumulación en el agua en ausencia de degradación. Sin embargo, esta posibilidad queda aparentemente excluida debido a la degradación por los microorganismos presentes en el suelo, los cienos de alcantarilla y el agua.

Las emisiones atmosféricas causadas por el uso de éteres glicólicos como solventes volátiles originan la máxima exposición ambiental. En el medio ambiente general, la degradación fotolítica parece ser rápida y cabe prever niveles inferiores a 0,0007 mg/m^3 (2 x 10^{-4} ppm).

En condiciones aeróbicas los microorganismos degradan rápidamente los éteres glicólicos en forma de dióxido de carbono y agua, mientras que en condiciones de anaerobiosis los principales productos finales son el metano y el dióxido de carbono.

4. Niveles en el medio ambiente y exposición humana

El uso de éteres glicólicos puede dar lugar a emisiones considerables y muy extendidas en el medio ambiente. Suscita especial preocupación la exposición humana directa en la industria, en los talleres de dimensiones modestas y como consecuencia del empleo doméstico de productos que contienen dichos éteres. Se han señalado valores de exposición profesional comprendidos entre < 0,1 mg/m^3 y > 150 mg/m^3. Los usuarios de productos de consumo pueden sufrir una exposición considerable, aunque no se dispone de datos al respecto.

Además de la exposición a los éteres glicólicos presentes en la atmósfera, las personas pueden estar expuestas por vía cutánea. Los análisis de sangre confirman que la absorción es rápida por esta vía, que puede contribuir más que la exposición atmosférica a la carga total que recibe el organismo.

5. Cinética y metabolismo

Se ha demostrado que los cuatro éteres glicólicos pueden absorberse rápidamente a través de la piel, los pulmones y el tracto gastrointestinal. Los valores más elevados que se han obtenido en los estudios sobre la distribución del 2-ME en ratonas gestantes se sitúan en el hígado, la sangre y el tracto gastrointestinal de la madre, así como en la placenta, el saco vitelino y en numerosas estructuras del embrión.

La transformación metabólica del 2-ME produce dos metabolitos primarios: MAA y glicina de 2-metoxiacetilo. La metabolización a dióxido de carbono representa una vía secundaria de menor importancia. La conversión del 2-ME en MAA en el plasma se produce rápidamente, con una vida media de 0,6 h en las ratas, pero la secreción del MAA es lenta, con una vida media de 20 h aproximadamente en la rata y de 77 h en el hombre.

En los animales de laboratorio, la administración de 2-EE da lugar a la producción de EAA y de glicina de 2-etoxiacetilo; el EAA es el principal metabolito que aparece en los testículos, que son el "órgano diana" presunto. En un estudio humano en el que se utilizó 2-EEA se observó una vía metabólica análoga: el acetato se hidrolizó primero en 2-EE y luego se transformó en EAA por oxidación. El EAA resultante se excretó con una vida media estimada en 21-42 h. Los estudios experimentales hacen pensar que la retención o acumulación de los metabolitos podrían ser importantes desde el punto de vista toxicológico en el supuesto de que dichos metabolitos sean la causa de la toxicidad observada en el "órgano diana".

6. Efectos en los organismos presentes en el medio ambiente

La toxicidad del 2-ME y del 2-EE para los microorganismos y animales acuáticos parece ser baja. En el caso de los microorganismos, la concentración letal en el medio es superior al 2%. Con el 2-ME se ha observado inhibición del crecimiento de las algas verdes a 10^4 mg/litro y de las cianobacterias (algas verde azuladas) a 100 mg/litro. La toxicidad aguda del 2-EE es muy baja para los artrópodos (CL_{50} > 4 g/litro) y para los peces de agua dulce

(CL_{50} > 10 g/litro). Los acetatos de éteres glicólicos (2-MEA y 2-EEA) son mucho más tóxicos para los peces. La CL_{50} del 2-EEA para el Phoxinus cabezudo es 46 mg/litro y la del 2-MEA para el pez plateado de la pleamar y los Lepomis de agallas azules es de 45 mg/litro. No se han hecho estudios a largo plazo.

7. Efectos en los animales de experimentación y en los sistemas de experimentación *in vitro*

7.1 Toxicidad sistémica

La toxicidad del 2-ME y del 2-EE en los animales de experimentación se ha estudiado en medida mucho mayor que la del 2-MA y del 2-EEA.

El 2-ME y el 2-EE y sus acetatos dan tasas análogas de letalidad tras una exposición única y producen una letalidad aguda baja cuando la exposición tiene lugar por vía dérmica u oral o por inhalación. Los valores de la DL_{50} oral en las diversas especies estudiadas oscilan entre 900 y 3400 mg/kg de peso corporal en el caso del 2-ME, entre 1400 y 5500 mg/kg en el del 2-EE, entre 1250 y 3930 mg/kg en el del 2-MEA, y entre 1300 y 5100 mg/kg en el de 2-EEA. En los ratones se han obtenido valores de la CL_{50} por inhalación de 4603 mg/m^3 (2-ME) y 6698 mg/m^3 (2-EE).

Sólo se dispone de datos limitados acerca de la irritación cutánea u ocular o del potencial de sensibilización de estos éteres glicólicos en los animales. Al parecer, no son irritantes para la piel, pero pueden causar irritación en los ojos. En el hombre no se ha observado irritación ni sensibilización cutáneas ni siquiera en caso de gran exposición.

La exposición por inhalación a corto plazo (hasta 90 días) de los animales de experimentación a concentraciones elevadas (> 9313 mg de 2-ME/m^3 y > 1450 mg de 2-EE/m^3) ejerce, según se ha demostrado, efectos adversos en los parámetros sanguíneos, el sistema nervioso y los testículos, el timo, el riñón, el hígado y los pulmones. Utilizando niveles más bajos de exposición, se han observado efectos en el sistema hematopoyético y en los testículos. Así, por ejemplo, las ratas expuestas durante 13 semanas a la inhalación de 2-ME a concentraciones comprendidas entre

93 y 930 mg/m^3 presentaron una reducción del volumen hematocrito y de los glóbulos blancos, la hemoglobina, las plaquetas y las concentraciones de proteínas séricas solamente cuando se aplicaba la dosis máxima, mientras que los ratones expuestos del mismo modo presentaron disminución del tamaño del timo además de la disminución de los parámetros sanguíneos con concentraciones de 930 mg/m^3. Las ratas y conejos expuestos al 2-EE presentaron efectos análogos pero menos intensos cuando soportaron durante 13 semanas una concentración de 1450 mg/m^3. No se dispone de datos sobre estudios a largo plazo.

7.2 Carcinogenicidad y mutagenicidad

La mutagenicidad del 2-ME se ha estudiado en una gama de sistemas in vitro utilizando bacterias y células de mamífero. Aunque la mayor parte de los estudios han dado resultados negativos, algunos informes acusan resultados positivos en cuanto a la mutagenicidad de las concentraciones muy altas de 2-ME en células CHO estudiadas desde el punto de vista de las aberraciones cromosómicas (a 6830 μg por ml o más) o del intercambio de cromátides equiparables (3170 μg/ml o más). En cambio, la investigación in vivo de aberraciones cromosómicas y micronúcleos ha dado siempre resultados negativos. Sólo se dispone de una información muy limitada sobre el potencial mutagénico del 2-EE y no se dispone de ningún dato sobre la carcinogenicidad de estos éteres glicólicos.

7.3 Sistema reproductor masculino

Los efectos del 2-ME en el sistema reproductor masculino se han estudiado detenidamente en roedores expuestos por vía oral o por inhalación. En el epitelio germinal de los tubos seminíferos se han observado constantemente alteraciones degenerativas. Análogos efectos se han obtenido con el 2-EE, si bien con niveles de dosificación algo más elevados.

En la rata, la administración oral de 2-ME durante 1-11 días ha dado lugar a un descenso del recuento de espermatozoides con cambios de la motilidad y la morfología de éstos en relación con la dosis utilizada; como niveles de dosificación se utilizaron 100 mg/kg de peso corporal o más. En la autopsia se encontraron acusadas alteraciones histológicas en los testículos. El nivel de efecto no observado (NENO) fue de 50 mg/kg. La reducción de la fertilidad seguía siendo patente a las 8 semanas de la exposición a 200 mg/kg. Análogos efectos se observaron con dosificaciones de 500 mg de 2-EE/kg o más, administrados durante 11 días como máximo; en el tratamiento de 11 días el NENO fue de 250 mg/kg. En cambio, cuando las reservas de espermatozoides están reducidas por la frecuencia de los acoplamientos, se observó cierta reducción de los recuentos con la dosis más baja estudiada. Los estudios de fertilidad consecutivos a la administración de una sola dosis oral de 250 mg de 2-ME/kg o más mostraron una esterilidad completa, tanto en las ratas como en los ratones, a partir de las 5 semanas de administración; con 125 mg/kg se observó ya cierto descenso de la fertilidad.

En los experimentos de inhalación se observaron alteraciones degenerativas análogas en los testículos con el 2-ME. Los efectos se observaron tras una sola exposición (4 h) a 1944 mg/m^3 o más pero no con 933 mg/m^3. El NENO fue de 311 mg/m^3 en la rata tras la exposición durante 13 semanas (6 h/día, 5 días/semana) y de 933 mg/m^3 (6 h/día) en los ratones tras la exposición en 9 ocasiones en el curso de 11 días. En los conejos expuestos al 2-ME durante 13 semanas (6 h/día, 5 días/semana) se observaron efectos marcados en los testículos con concentraciones de 311 mg/m^3 o más y efectos marginales con 93 mg/m^3; no se determinó el NENO.

7.4 Toxicidad para el desarrollo

En varias especies de animales de laboratorio se ha observado toxicidad para el desarrollo tras la exposición a los compuestos utilizando todas las vías de administración: oral, inhalatoria y dérmica. El 2-ME produjo efectos teratógenos en ratones, ratas, conejos y monos. El 2-EE y el 2-EEA resultaron teratógenos en las ratas y los ratones. Aunque no se ha estudiado la toxicidad sobre el desarrollo del 2-MEA, los perfiles metabólicos (véase la sección 6) hacen pensar que es posible que el 2-MEA tenga una toxicidad análoga a la del 2-ME.

En relación con el 2-ME se dispone de la gama más amplia de datos dosis/respuesta (dosis de 31,25 por 1000 mg/kg por día). En este estudio de administración intensiva en el que se utilizaron ratones (2-ME administrado entre el 7° y el 14° día de gestación) el NENO correspondiente a la toxicidad materna fue de 125 mg/kg por día. No obstante, se observaron malformaciones con 62,5 mg/kg por día y variaciones esqueléticas con 31,25 mg/kg por día. No se señaló ningún NENO de toxicidad para el desarrollo. En el marco de estudios de dosis única, se trató a ratones con 2-ME administrado por alimentación forzada el 11° día de la gestación; la dosis de 100 mg/kg no era fetotóxica mientras que la de 175 mg/kg produjo anomalías digitales sin otros signos de toxicidad materna o fetal. En la ratas recién nacidas se observaron defectos cardiovasculares y anomalías del ECG tras el tratamiento de las madres con 25 mg/kg por día durante los días 7° a 13° de la gestación. Como ésta fue la dosis más baja que se ensayó, este estudio no ha permitido establecer un NENO para el desarrollo (con esa dosis no se observó toxicidad materna). De igual modo, no pudo determinarse ningún NENO de toxicidad para el desarrollo en un estudio de tratamiento de monos por alimentación forzada con 2-ME a 0,16, 0,32 o 0,47 mmol/kg por día durante los días 20° a 45° de la gestación.

Tras la exposición a la inhalación de 2-ME a 156 mg por m³ se ha observado fetotoxicidad en los ratones y ratas y malformaciones en los conejos. En las tres especies, el NENO correspondiente a los efectos sobre el desarrollo fue de 31 mg/m³. Sin embargo, en la descendencia de las ratas expuestas a 78 mg 2-ME/m³ durante los días 7-13 o 14-20 de la gestación se observaron alteraciones conductuales y neuroquímicas.

Tras la exposición por inhalación de ratas (743 mg por m³) y conejos (589 mg/m³), el 2-EE se reveló teratógeno (en presencia de ligera toxicidad materna). En otro estudio se observó fetotoxicidad pero no malformaciones en las ratas expuestas a 184 ó 920 mg de 2-EE/m³, así como en los conejos expuestos a 644 mg de 2-EE/m³. Los valores del NENO para los efectos en el desarrollo fueron de 37 mg/m³ en las ratas y de 184 mg/m³ en los conejos. En la descendencia de las ratas expuestas a 368 mg de 2-EE por m³ durante los días 7-13 ó 14-20 de la gestación se observaron alteraciones conductuales y neuroquímicas.

Las ratas tratadas por aplicación dérmica de 0,25 ml de 2-EE sin diluir (cuatro veces al día en los días 7-16 de la gestación) acusaron una considerable fetotoxicidad y una elevada incidencia de malformaciones en ausencia de toxicidad materna. Análogos efectos se observaron tras el tratamiento de las ratas con 2-EEA, utilizando el mismo protocolo, a una dosis equimolar (0,35 ml, cuatro veces al día).

La exposición por inhalación de 2-EEA de conejas durante los días 6-18 de la gestación provocó respuestas teratógenas con 2176 mg/m^3 y 544 mg/m^3 en dos estudios diferentes, en los cuales los valores del NENO para el desarrollo fueron de 135 mg/m^3 y 270 mg/m^3. Las ratas expuestas al 2-EEA durante los días 6-15 de la gestación acusaron fetotoxicidad a 540 mg/m^3 y malformaciones a 1080 mg/m^3. El NENO para el desarrollo fue de 170 mg por m^3.

8. Efectos en el hombre

La información disponible sobre los efectos tóxicos de estos cuatro éteres glicólicos en el ser humano es limitada. Los resultados de los escasos informes sobre casos individuales y estudios epidemiológicos en el lugar de trabajo corroboran los efectos adversos observados en los animales de experimentación. No se ha encontrado ningún informe en el que se cuantifique la exposición y los efectos adversos en la población general.

En dos casos no mortales de envenenamiento por ingestión de 100 ml de 2-ME, los signos y síntomas predominantes fueron náuseas, vértigo, cianosis, taquicardia, hiperventilación y acidosis metabólica, con algunos indicios de insuficiencia renal. Síntomas análogos, aunque menos graves, se observaron en un sujeto que ingirió 40 ml de 2-EE. En un caso de intoxicación mortal causada por la ingestión de 400 ml de 2-ME, la autopsia reveló una gastritis hemorrágica aguda con degeneración grasa del hígado y alteraciones degenerativas de los túbulos renales.

La exposición repetida de los trabajadores al 2-ME y al 2-EE, así como a otros solventes, ha dado lugar a anemia, leucopenia, debilidad general y ataxia. En muchos de estos estudios no se ha hecho ninguna estimación fidedigna de la exposición. Los efectos hematológicos de los éteres glicólicos en el ser humano están bien documentados y se ha descrito la aparición de anemia macrocítica en un trabajador expuesto al 2-ME (promedio: 105 mg/m^3), así como a otros solventes.

En los trabajadores expuestos por vía dérmica al 2-ME se han observado efectos tóxicos en la médula ósea, y también se han observado efectos inmunológicos en trabajadores sometidos a una exposición prolongada (8-35 años) al 2-ME y al 2-EE (los promedios de exposición fueron de 6,1 mg/m^3 y 4,8 mg/m^3, respectivamente).

Los estudios epidemiológicos realizados en trabajadores expuestos al 2-ME y al 2-EE han revelado algunos indicios de efectos adversos en el sistema reproductor masculino, con un aumento de la frecuencia de recuentos reducidos de espermatozoides. La exposición al 2-EE (37 trabajadores) a concentraciones de hasta 88,5 mg/m^3 provocaron una alteración de los índices seminales. En un grupo de 73 trabajadores expuestos al 2-ME (hasta 17,7 mg por m^3) y al 2-EE (hasta 80,5 mg/m^3) se observó una mayor frecuencia de recuentos reducidos de espermatozoides y también signos de efectos hematológicos con exposiciones de 2,6 mg/m^3 para el 2-ME y de 9,9 mg/m^3 para el 2-EE (TWA).

Los efectos adversos observados en las personas profesionalmente expuestas coinciden con los señalados en los animales de experimentación. Sin embargo, debido a deficiencias en las evaluaciones de la exposición y a las exposiciones mixtas, no se han podido determinar relaciones dosis-respuesta.

9. Conclusiones

Muchas personas pueden estar expuestas a concentraciones de estos cuatro éteres glicólicos comparables a las industriales a consecuencia del empleo de productos comerciales y de consumo. Tanto por inhalación como por absorción cutánea pueden producirse exposiciones profesionales importantes. En un número limitado de determinaciones de la concentración atmosférica en los lugares de trabajo se han obtenido valores comprendidos entre < 0,1 mg/m^3 y > 150 mg/m^3.

Tanto el 2-ME como el 2-EE se muestran poco tóxicos para los microorganismos y las especies acuáticas. No se dispone de datos que permitan precisar la capacidad potencial de las exposiciones prolongadas para ejercer efectos adversos sobre las especies presentes en el medio ambiente.

En las ratas se ha obtenido un NENO para los efectos testiculares de 933 mg de 2-ME/m^3, así como un NENO para la exposición repetida de 311 mg/m^3. En los experimentos de exposición repetida con la especie más sensible, el conejo, se ha detectado un efecto neto con 311 mg/m^3, mientras que a 93 mg/m^3 se observaba un efecto marginal (1 de 5 animales). En las personas expuestas profesionalmente al 2-ME y al 2-EE se han encontrado indicios de que estos éteres glicólicos pueden producir toxicidad testicular en el ser humano.

En todas las especies (ratones, ratas y conejos) expuestas al 2-ME a 156 mg/m^3 o más se ha observado toxicidad para el desarrollo. Para las tres especies se tuvo un NENO de 31 mg/m^3. En las ratas expuestas in utero a 78 mg/m^3 se produjeron alteraciones conductuales y neuroquímicas, pero no se estableció ningún valor de NENO. El 2-EE y el 2-EEA eran algo menos potentes. En la rata y en el conejo se han observado efectos sobre el desarrollo tras la exposición a 2-EE a concentraciones de 368 mg por m^3 o más. Estos efectos eran ligeros en las ratas expuestas a 184 mg de 2-EE/m^3, pero tanto en las ratas como en los conejos se pudo establecer un NENO bien definido a 37 mg/m^3.

Estos éteres glicólicos producen efectos hematológicos en los ratones, las ratas, los conejos, los perros, los hamsters, y los cobayos. Esta observación concuerda con los efectos hematológicos señalados en algunos de los escasos estudios efectuados en trabajadores industriales expuestos repetidamente al 2-EE y/o al 2-ME. En los estudios de exposición repetida de animales se obtuvo un NENO de 93 mg de 2-ME/m^3 en los conejos y de 368 mg de 2-EE por m^3 en las ratas y los conejos. No se han obtenido datos que permitan evaluar cuantitativamente los efectos hematológicos que siguen a la exposición aguda.

EVALUACION DE LOS RIESGOS PARA LA SALUD HUMANA Y EFECTOS EN EL MEDIO AMBIENTE

1. Evaluación de los riesgos para la salud humana

1.1 Exposición

Muchas personas pueden estar expuestas al 2-metoxietanol (2-ME), al 2-etoxietanol (2-EE) y a sus acetatos (2-MEA y 2-EEA) en concentraciones comparables a las industriales como consecuencia del empleo de productos comerciales y de consumo. En cambio, la exposición por los alimentos, el agua o el aire ambiente es probablemente insignificante. Esta impresión se basa únicamente en las propiedades físicas y químicas de estos compuestos y en los indicios de que experimentan una rápida degradación en el medio ambiente.

Tanto por inhalación como por absorción cutánea puede producirse una exposición profesional importante. Las escasas determinaciones de las concentraciones en la atmósfera de los lugares de trabajo han dado valores comprendidos entre menos de 0,1 mg/m^3 y más de 150 mg por m^3. Sin embargo, las posibilidades de vigilancia son muy limitadas y cabe la posibilidad de que haya grandes variaciones entre diferentes industrias e incluso dentro de una misma industria. Habida cuenta de las posibilidades de absorción cutánea, la vigilancia del aire por sí sola puede dar una subestimación de la exposición total. La vigilancia biológica es el mejor método para calcular la absorción total. Entre los trabajos que entrañan una exposición considerable figuran, por ejemplo, los de pintura, imprenta y limpieza; ahora bien, no hay que olvidar que estos compuestos se utilizan también en otras muchas actividades profesionales en las que la exposición debe ser motivo de inquietud.

1.2 Efectos en la salud

Los principales motivos de inquietud en el ser humano son los efectos en el desarrollo, los efectos testiculares y los vinculados a la toxicidad hematológica. Estos efectos han sido demostrados por una multitud de datos sólidos obtenidos en el animal y por algunos datos de origen humano. Todos ellos pueden estar causados por una exposición a corto o a largo plazo. En los animales de experimentación, la exposición muy repetida al 2-ME y al 2-EE (más de 939 y 1450 mg/m^3, respectivamente) produce efectos tóxicos neuroconductuales, hepáticos y renales, los cuales se observan también en casos de intoxicación humana.

Estos cuatro éteres glicólicos dan valores muy similares de toxicidad testicular y de toxicidad para el desarrollo en todas las especies estudiadas y por todas las vías de exposición que se han ensayado (inhalatoria, dérmica y oral). En los estudios sobre el mecanismo de acción se ha visto que la metabolización al derivado del ácido alcoxiacético constituye una etapa indispensable de activación, tanto en los efectos sobre el desarrollo como en los testiculares. Dicho metabolismo se efectúa mediante el sistema de deshidrogenasa alcohólica que es común al hombre y a los animales de laboratorio. Los metabolitos tóxicos, el ácido metoxiacético (MAA) y el ácido etoxi-acético (EAA), aparecen en la orina de las personas expuestas a estos solventes. La coherencia de las respuestas en las distintas especies de animales de laboratorio estudiadas, junto con la semejanza del metabolismo en el ser humano, permiten concluir que el hombre está probablemente expuesto a los efectos testiculares y sobre el desarrollo de estos éteres glicólicos. Los datos disponibles sobre la excreción de ácidos alcoxiacéticos por el hombre sugieren la existencia de una retención prolongada en comparación con la que se observa en los animales de laboratorio, lo cual hace pensar que las personas quizás sean más sensibles que las especies experimentales de mayor sensibilidad. Un motivo de especial inquietud es la rápida absorción cutánea de estos compuestos. Se han observado efectos teratógenos y otros efectos sobre el desarrollo tras la aplicación de 2-ME, 2-EE y 2-EEA en la piel intacta de la rata.

En la rata, el ratón y el conejo se han observado alteraciones testiculares tras la exposición a estos éteres glicólicos, tanto por inhalación como por vía oral. Una exposición aislada de la rata a la inhalación de 1944 mg de 2-ME/m^3 o más durante 4 h y la exposición repetida a 933 mg de 2-ME/m^3 o más durante 13 semanas han provocado signos histológicos evidentes de alteración testicular. El NENO para la exposición aguda fue de 933 mg/m^3 y para la exposición repetida de 311 mg/m^3. El ratón parece ser menos sensible, siendo el NENO para la exposición repetida de 933 mg/m^3. En cambio, el conejo resulta más sensible, observándose en él alteraciones testiculares marcadas tras la exposición repetida a 311 mg/m^3 y un efecto marginal (uno en cinco conejos afectados) a 93 mg por m^3. Efectos análogos se han observado tras la exposición oral de la rata al 2-ME, con aparición de lesiones testiculares tras la exposición breve (inclusive de dosis única) a 100 mg/kg. En un estu-dio subagudo (11 días) el NENO fue de 50 mg/kg. El 2-EE es algo menos potente respecto a la toxicidad testicular que el 2-ME; sólo se observaron efectos con dosificaciones de 500 mg/kg o más, siendo el NENO de 250 mg/kg.

Los datos obtenidos en las personas profesionalmente expuestas al 2-ME y al 2-EE coinciden con los de los estudios en animales e indican que estos éteres glicólicos pueden producir toxicidad testicular en el ser humano. Los estudios epidemiológicos de pequeños grupos de trabajadores expuestos al 2-EE en una empresa de fundición de metales y de pintores de embarcaciones expuestos tanto al 2-ME como al 2-EE muestran indefectiblemente una mayor incidencia de recuentos reducidos de espermatozoides. Los datos sobre los niveles de exposición, aunque limitados, aportan en cada caso pruebas de la exposición dérmica así como de la exposición por inhalación.

En la rata, el ratón, el conejo y el mono se han observado efectos tóxicos sobre el desarrollo tras la exposición a estos éteres glicólicos por vía dérmica, oral o inhalatoria. Con 12 aplicaciones diarias de 2-ME sin diluir en la piel rasurada de ratas gestantes (oclusión: 6 h) se obtuvo un efecto letal, mientras que 10 aplicaciones abiertas de 2-EE (1,0 ml/día) o 2-EEA (1,4 ml/día) se mostraron teratógenas pero no tóxicas para la madre. Doce aplicaciones cerradas de 2-ME al 10% en suero salino resultaron tóxicas para el desarrollo (en este estudio el NENO fue del 3% para el 2-ME. No se han encontrado niveles sin efecto aparente tras la administración oral repetida de 2-ME a las hembras preñadas. El nivel de efecto observado mínimo (NEOM) en la administración oral de 2-ME fue de 31,25 mg/kg por día en el caso de los ratones, de 25 mg por kg por día en el de las ratas y de 0,16 mmol/kg por día en el de los monos. Sólo se han hecho experimentos de dosis única con el 2-ME en los ratones, con el resultado de que el 11° día de la gestación (que es el día más sensible) el NENO era de 100 mg/kg y el NEOM de 175 mg/kg. Tanto el 2-EE como el 2-EEA se han evaluado en ratas y conejos por inhalación. A las ratas se las expuso al 2-EE en dos estudios, en los que se obtuvieron efectos teratógenos (743 mg/m^3 durante 7 h/día los días 1-19 de la gestación) o efectos fetotóxicos (184 y 920 mg/m^3 durante 6 h por día los días 6-15 de la gestación). En este último estudio, el NENO fue de 37 mg/m^3. También los conejos expuestos al 2-EE presentaron efectos teratógenos (589 mg por m^3 durante 7 h/día los días 1-18 de la gestación) o efectos fetotóxicos (644 mg/m^3 durante 6 h/día los días 6-18 de la gestación). En el último estudio, el NENO fue de 184 mg/m^3. En los conejos expuestos al 2-EEA durante 6 h/día los días 6-18 de la gestación se obtuvieron efectos teratógenos a 2160 mg/m^3 en un estudio y a 1620 mg por m^3 en otro. En ambos estudios se observó fetotoxicidad a 540 mg/m^3 y en uno y otro el nivel de exposición mínimo (135 y 270 mg/m^3, respectivamente) coincidía con el NENO. Las ratas expuestas al 2-EEA por inhalación durante 6 h/día los días 6-15 de la gestación presentaron el mismo tipo de expuesta: efectos teratógenos a 1620 mg por m^3, fetotoxicidad a 1080 mg/m^3 y ausencia de todo efecto a 270 mg/m^3.

Así, pues, se ha observado toxicidad para el desarrollo en todas las especies (ratones, ratas y conejos) expuestas al 2-ME a 156 mg/m^3 o más. Para las tres especies, el NENO fue de 31 mg/m^3. En ratas expuestas *in utero* a 78 mg/m^3 se han observado alteraciones conductuales y neuroquímicas, no habiéndose señalado ningún NENO.

El 2-EE y el 2-EEA han resultado algo menos potentes. En la rata y el conejo, todas las exposiciones al 2-EE a 368 mg/m^3 o más fueron seguidas de efectos sobre el desarrollo. En las ratas expuestas a 184 mg de 2-EE/m^3 estos efectos eran leves, pero 37 mg/m^3 constituía un NENO patente. En el caso del 2-EEA, el NENO era de 170 mg/m^3 tanto en la rata como en el conejo.

Tanto en los animales como en los casos de envenenamiento humano se han observado efectos hematológicos tras la exposición a una dosis aguda única. La exposición por inhalación repetida de la especie más sensible, el conejo, al 2-ME durante 13 semanas y a razón de cinco veces por semana dio un NEI de 93 mg/m^3. También las dosis repetidas de 2-ME provocan toxicidad hematológica en los ratones, conejos, perros, hámsters y cobayos. El 2-EE es menos potente que el 2-ME como causa de efectos hematológicos. El NENO correspondiente a estos efectos fue de 368 mg/m^3 en las ratas y los conejos expuestos a 2-EE durante 13 semanas a razón de cinco veces por semana durante 6 h/día. También en los perros y los ratones se han registrado efectos hematológicos tras la exposición repetida a concentraciones más elevadas de 2-EE. La exposición a los ésteres acéticos del 2-EE y del 2-ME quizá provoque efectos análogos a los mismos niveles de exposición, pero los datos disponibles sobre exposición y efectos hematológicos de esos compuestos son demasiado escasos para determinar en qué condiciones una exposición humana aislada tendrá efectos hematológicos.

Se han observado niveles de exposición industrial próximos o idénticos al NENO de efectos hematológicos en animales expuestos a dosis repetidas de 2-ME o de 2-EE. Este hecho, junto con la mayor sensibilidad que probablemente tienen las personas y la acumulación previsible de metabolitos en la sangre humana, hace pensar que tanto la exposición industrial como la de los consumidores pueden tener efectos hematológicos. Esto ha sido confirmado por la observación de efectos de este tipo en algunos de los escasos estudios realizados sobre trabajadores industriales expuestos repetidamente al 2-EE, al 2-ME o a ambos compuestos a la vez.

2. Evaluación de los efectos sobre el medio ambiente

La exposición ambiental a estos éteres glicólicos puede producirse como consecuencia de su paso directo a la atmósfera cuando se utilizan como solventes volátiles. También pueden ser causa de exposición ambiental los vertidos en el suelo y el agua a consecuencia de escapes accidentales. La acumulación en el suelo y en las aguas superficiales sólo podría producirse en ausencia de degradación. Sin embargo, estos éteres glicólicos se degradan rápidamente a causa de procesos químicos y biológicos, por lo que no es probable que se acumulen. Tanto el 2-MEA como el 2-EEA pueden hidrolizarse fácilmente y, por consiguiente, biodegradarse en condiciones aerobias. En cambio, la contaminación de acuíferos y suelos anaerobios sigue planteando un problema potencial, aunque es de esperar que no pase de ser una situación transitoria y, por ende, poco peligrosa.

Tanto el 2-ME como el 2-EE se muestran poco tóxicos con los microorganismos y las especies acuáticas. Los acetatos de éteres glicólicos, en cambio, tienen una toxicidad aguda mucho mayor. No se dispone de datos para calcular las posibilidades de efectos adversos en especies del medio ambiente a causa de la exposición prolongada.

RECOMENDACIONES

1. Protección de la salud

1. Hay que identificar otros solventes menos tóxicos que puedan sustituir al 2-metoxietanol, al 2-etoxietanol y a sus ésteres, especialmente en los productos destinados al consumo. También es particularme importante evaluar los efectos de otros éteres etilenglicólicos, ya que algunos pueden tener efectos análogos a los de los cuatro éteres glicólicos que aquí se evalúan.

2. Habida cuenta de los conocidos efectos tóxicos de estos éteres glicólicos, las autoridades deben ocuparse seriamente de establecer estrategias apropiadas para informar a los usuarios de esos productos acerca de los riesgos que entrañan, especialmente los resultantes de la exposición dérmica.

3. En vista de los nuevos datos toxicológicos y de las posibilidades de absorción dérmica importante de estos éteres glicólicos, habrá que reconsiderar los límites de exposición profesional fijados por los países a fin de que la dosis diaria total que reciben los trabajadores por todas las vías de administración no plantee un riesgo indebido para la salud.

4. En los animales se observan efectos de dosis única en niveles de exposición bastante altos. Con objeto de reducir los riesgos para la salud, se recomienda utilizar con prudencia estos compuestos (prestando atención a la higiene personal, los dispositivos apropiados de protección y la ventilación adecuada). Los datos disponibles indican que puede ser necesario aumentar la protección a fin de evitar efectos en el desarrollo, así como en la sangre y los testículos como resultando de la exposición repetida.

2. Investigaciones necesarias

1. En vista de la intervención del ácido metoxiacético (MAA) y etoxiacético (EAA) (que son los principales metabolitos identificados del 2-ME, del 2-EE y de sus ésteres) en la toxicidad para el sistema reproductor masculino,

habrá que investigar su mecanismo de acción. Si de ello se deduce que el MAA y el EAA no son los principales agentes responsables, habrá que tratar de identificar éstos y de aclarar su mecanismo de acción.

2. Estos cuatro éteres glicólicos tienen a la vez efectos hematológicos y efectos sobre el sitema reproductor masculino (reducción del recuento de espermatozoides). Los datos disponibles, aunque limitados, parecen indicar que ambos efectos se hacen evidentes a niveles de dosificación análogos. Habrá que investigar el mecanismo de acción en ambos sistemas orgánicos y examinar paralelamente los efectos hematológicos y los recuentos de espermatozoides con el fin de determinar si las alteraciones de la sangre proporcionan signos de alarma con repecto a otros efectos de estos compuestos.

3. La vigilancia del aire no basta por sí sola para garantizar una exposición de poca intensidad. La vigilancia biológica puede contribuir a detectar defectos de las medidas de protección. De momento no se ha establecido claramente la relación existente entre los indicadores biológicos de exposición, la absorción corporal total y los efectos observados en la salud. Habrá que proseguir las investigaciones a fin de adquirir una base para aplicar la vigilancia biológica a la determinación de la seguridad en las exposiciones.

4. Hay que proyectar estudios epidemiológicos y/o trabajos específicos de vigilancia sanitaria en poblaciones muy expuestas a estos éteres glicólicos a fin de estimar las relaciones exposición-efecto con miras a determinar exposiciones seguras, siempre que se pueda evaluar adecuada y suficientemente la exposición total mediante la vigilancia ambiental y biológica.

5. Habrá que investigar la posibilidad de que estos compuestos ejerzan efectos sobre las gónadas femeninas mediante estudios de reproducción multigeneracional en animales.

6. Los datos disponibles indican que el ser humano puede metabolizar estos éteres glicólicos hasta los correspondientes ácidos alcoxiacéticos en mayor medida que la rata, y que la vida media de la excreción urinaria de estos metabolitos tóxicos es aproximadamente cuatro veces más

prolongada en las personas que en las ratas. Por otra parte, éstas conjugan una mayor cantidad de los metabolitos ácidos, cosa que no hacen las personas. Estas diferencias podrían explicar la sensibilidad relativamente elevada del ser humano a estos éteres glicólicos. Un conocimiento detallado del metabolismo y de la cinética de excreción mejoraría nuestra capacidad para predecir cuáles son los niveles de exposición seguros.

7. Los resultados obtenidos en estudios a corto plazo (13 semanas) indican efectos en diversos sistemas orgánicos. En cambio, no se han hecho estudios de suficiente duración que permitan evaluar la reversibilidad de tales efectos. Por consiguiente, convendría que se emprendieran estudios de interrupción en los que los animales de experimentación estuvieran expuestos a estos éteres glicólicos al menos durante 13 semanas, seguidas de un periodo apropiado de recuperación. Cabría evaluar así importantes parámetros fisiológicos con miras a determinar si esos efectos son o no transitorios.